Contents

Introduction

Let's say it up front: Diabetes is incurable. Despite all the advancements that have been made in medical science over the past fifty years, there is still no cure for diabetes.

However, that doesn't mean that there isn't anything positive to say about diabetes treatment. The fact is that diabetes is manageable. In fact, with the right medical treatment and diligent self-management, most people with diabetes live active, full, and productive lives. Even more important, if diabetes is managed properly, people with diabetes can expect their length of life to be normal.

There is also good news about preventing diabetes. New evidence suggests that some cases of diabetes can be prevented by simply losing weight, lowering one's cholesterol, and keeping physically active. And prevention is more in the spotlight these days as we see the number of new cases of diabetes steadily grow each year.

There are close to sixteen million Americans with diabetes. And shockingly, close to six million of those people have not been diagnosed. This latter group is a serious problem.

Without proper diagnosis and treatment, they are likely to be the people who suffer all the terrible side effects of diabetes—from blindness to early death. Also alarming is the fact that the number of diabetics is growing. Between 1993 and 1997, the numbers increased by two million people. This growth suggests a very strong lifestyle connection.

Understanding diabetes, how to help prevent it, and how to treat it is a key to taking control of your own health. And that is exactly why we have written this book. In the pages that follow, we present the most up-do-date information available about diabetes. Our purpose is to help you in making all the important lifestyle and treatment decisions that confront a person with diabetes.

While diagnosed by a physician and usually managed by medical personnel, diabetes treatment is primarily self-care. That means the more you know about the disease and the options you have, the better able you will be to treat yourself. It is important that you know about the breakthroughs that have occurred in diabetes treatment in just the past few years. For example, there is a new form of insulin that works more quickly. And people who use therapy that closely controls blood-sugar levels may reduce their risk of developing eye problems, kidney disease, and other diabetic complications by 50 to 70 percent.

As the nation's foremost nonprofit consumer health advocacy organization, the People's Medical Society is dedicated to empowering the medical consumer. Study upon study confirms that the more you know about your condition, the more likely it is to be under control. And the more you understand your options, the more likely you are to be a strong partner with your health care providers.

This book is a key to your personal health empowerment. Remember the good news about diabetes—it's treatable. But also remember that the success of that treatment rests primarily with you. So the more you know, the more likely you are to live a normal and active life.

Charles B. Inlander
President
People's Medical Society

CHAPTER ONE

Diagnosis: Diabetes

DIABETES IS A SERIOUS DISEASE. IT IS CHRONIC, WHICH MEANS THAT it does not go away. If left unchecked, diabetes can shorten life.

That's the bad news.

But there's good news: Despite the fact that the causes of diabetes remain somewhat of a mystery, its treatment is far from unknown. Once you know you have diabetes, you can learn to take steps to control it. In *Understanding Diabetes*, you can find plenty of hands-on information about managing diabetes, and we guide you to additional resources. With such information, many people with diabetes have taken personal responsibility for managing their disease and, as a result, live normal, productive lives.

If you have diabetes, you should realize you're not alone. In the world, it is estimated that well over 100 million people have diabetes. In the United States, an estimated 15.7 million people are affected by the disease—and that includes people of all ages, from children to the elderly. And this number increases yearly; in 1997, the Centers for Disease Control and Prevention (CDC) reported the number of Americans with diabetes had increased sixfold over the past forty years, and in 1998, the American Diabetes Association reported that the incidence of type 2 diabetes increased by 9 percent per year between 1987 and 1996. Researchers attribute the increase to the increasing age of the American population and the fact that Americans get less physical activity and eat more fatty foods than ever before.

Each day, 2,200 cases of diabetes are diagnosed. Despite that staggering figure, diabetes all too often goes undiagnosed: The American Diabetes Association estimates that of the 15.7 million Americans with diabetes, 5.4 million have the condition but don't know it.

It may seem hard to believe that a disease as serious as diabetes could go unrecognized. But that's not so surprising when you take into account that diabetes comes on slowly: Scientists estimate that the disease may begin developing anywhere from four to twelve years before it is diagnosed. That means someone may have diabetes five, eight, even ten years before it's detected, depending upon the kind of diabetes that person has. Unfortunately, the condition can damage the body in that time, and many people only find out about their diabetes once they're having trouble with their eyes, nerves, kidneys, blood vessels, or heart.

What Is Diabetes?

Diabetes is a malfunction in the body's ability to convert carbohydrates—sweet and starchy foods, such as fruit, bread, and vegetables—into energy to power the body. The medical name for diabetes is **diabetes mellitus,** meaning "honey-sweet diabetes." As you might gather from such a name, diabetes is characterized by an abnormally high and persistent concentration of sugar in the bloodstream that doctors refer to as "elevated **plasma glucose.**" People affected with diabetes generally require lifelong medical care to control the disease.

Although by definition diabetes is a malfunction linked to carbohydrates, the problem is not so much the carbohydrates per se, but the way the body uses them to create energy. The process of converting food into energy is called **metabolism,** and diabetes is often called a metabolic disorder.

To explain why carbohydrates pose a problem, let's look first at the metabolic system of a healthy person.

Typically, in the body carbohydrates are converted to glucose and other simple sugars in the stomach and small intestine. Glucose moves from these organs into the blood vessels.

Spotting the Symptoms

Diabetes symptoms can be hard to pinpoint. In fact, sometimes there may not be any symptoms at all. But if you're looking for a rough guideline on what to look for, here's what the medical literature mentions as important symptoms of untreated or inadequately treated diabetes. We refer to these symptoms often through this chapter and the rest of the book:

Polyuria: This is the passing of too much urine, or frequent urination, as the kidneys strive to eliminate excess sugar.

Thirst: As you might suspect, polyuria causes dehydration, which, in turn, causes thirst.

Weight loss: The loss of water through frequent urination causes weight loss. Further contributing to weight loss is the need for the body to use **protein** and fat to supply the energy that normally would be supplied by properly metabolized glucose.

Tiredness is often present in diabetes, but is not considered a sure symptom because it can be associated with many other disorders. Other symptoms include unrelenting hunger, itching of the genitals and skin, visual disturbances (such as blurry vision), skin disorders (for example, boils), and pain and/or numbness of the extremities.

The blood circulates glucose through the body, carrying it to liver, muscle, and fat cells. Once the glucose reaches those cells, the hormone **insulin** enables it to be absorbed into the cells, either to be stored for later use or to be used immediately as energy. Thus, glucose powers the muscles, heart, and brain and assists the body in maintaining a constant temperature.

The body of a person with diabetes also converts carbohydrates to sugars and sends them into the blood. But at this point, the system comes to a crashing halt: The glucose is unable to enter the cells because of a lack of insulin in the body.

Insulin comes from the **pancreas**—a six-inch-long gland that is located behind the stomach. In healthy people, the pancreas secretes many fluids, including insulin. However, in a person with diabetes, one of two things happens: No insulin—or not enough insulin—is produced, or what the pancreas does produce does not function properly. In either case, the system has gone awry. Insulin alone enables the cells to absorb glucose for use as energy, and without it, a "glucose glut" eventually results—high levels of unused blood sugar are trapped in the bloodstream.

High blood sugar is a health risk. As sugar builds in the bloodstream, the kidneys try to filter it out. To eliminate the sugar, the kidneys must dissolve it. The more sugar there is to be eliminated, the more urine that must be passed.

You can see how this situation quickly leads to frequent urination and increased thirst—two of the symptoms of diabetes. Although the kidneys effectively keep the body from becoming overrun with sugar, working double time wears out the kidneys earlier than normal. Over a lifetime, such overwork eventually brings on kidney failure.

But that's not the only problem with high blood sugar. At the same time that the kidneys are furiously flushing the system of sugar, the body is seriously low on fuel. The body's cells, unable to burn sugar, begin to use protein and body fat as sources of energy.

This breakdown of fats for fuel releases toxic acids called **ketones.** Some ketones are excreted through the urine. Eventually, however, the ketones accumulate, and at high levels they can lead to a condition called **ketoacidosis,** which is in effect a poisoning of the system. Initial symptoms of this are frequent urination, increased thirst and dry mouth, the latter a result of dehydration. In extreme cases, ketoacidosis can cause unconsciousness—what some people call a **diabetic coma.** If left untreated, ketoacidosis can kill.

In nearly all situations, people with diabetes require, at a minimum, routine medical treatment, including daily self-care. For some people, this means taking insulin; for others, it means losing weight; for some, it means both. For all people with diabetes, it means paying particular attention to diet and exercise—what we mean by a lifestyle change.

The Dangers of Diabetes

The very nature of diabetes puts the sufferer at risk for serious complications; some experts believe the condition is now the nation's third or fourth leading cause of death. If diabetes goes unchecked, it will hasten wear and tear on many crucial bodily functions. In particular, it attacks:

The circulatory system. According to the American Diabetes Association, diabetes leads to coronary heart disease, stroke, and circulation problems in the hands and feet. These conditions are two to four times more common in people with diabetes, and they account for most of their hospitalizations. Heart attacks, hardening of the arteries, strokes, poor circulation in the feet, amputations—these are specific and common examples of diabetes damage.

The kidneys. Diabetes is the leading cause of kidney failure.

The eyes. Diabetic eye disease, or **diabetic retinopathy,** is the major cause of newly occurring vision loss in Americans twenty to seventy-four years old, according to the National Eye Institute.

The nervous system. Nerve cells may be disturbed or damaged, causing severe pain or loss of feeling that often begins in the arms and the legs—a condition known as **neuropathy.**

continues

We examine in detail the complications of diabetes in Chapter 4, but this illustrates the reasons that the condition must be treated seriously.

Types of Diabetes

Although people tend to think of diabetes as one disease, it really is a group of disorders. What they all have in common is a problem with insulin production or insulin action. Although a number of conditions are considered types of diabetes, the two most common disorders are type 1 diabetes and type 2 diabetes. You may also see these written with Roman numerals, as type I and type II diabetes. However, in 1997, the U.S. Committee on the Diagnosis and Classification of Diabetes Mellitus recommended that Arabic numbers be used to avoid confusion between the Roman numeral II and the number 11.

TYPE 1 DIABETES

Type 1 diabetes is the most severe form of diabetes. People with type 1 diabetes generally depend on injections of insulin to regulate their sugar metabolism. For this reason, the condition was also once called **insulin-dependent diabetes.** However, experts now identify the condition only as type 1 diabetes in a move away from basing the name of the condition on its treatment.

In the past, type 1 diabetes was also called **juvenile diabetes** because doctors thought that it would strike only children or young adults. Doctors now know that people of any age can develop type 1 diabetes, although the majority of cases are discovered in people younger than twenty.

People with type 1 diabetes are vulnerable to dangerous short-term complications of the disease. Two of these complications have to do with disruptive swings in blood-sugar levels, such as **hyperglycemia** (too much blood sugar) and **hypoglycemia** (too little blood sugar). People with type 1 diabetes also are at particular risk of ketoacidosis, that dangerous buildup of toxic acids in the body that we mentioned earlier.

Almost all Caucasian diabetic children (Caucasian children develop the condition much more frequently than children of other racial groups) and about 10 percent of adult diabetics have type 1, according to George S. Eisenbarth, M.D., of the Joslin Diabetes Center in Falmouth, Massachusetts, and Harvard Medical School. All this translates into big numbers: An estimated 500,000 to 1 million Americans have type 1 diabetes.

Experts call type 1 diabetes an **autoimmune** disease and suggest that it is genetically programmed. (*Autoimmune* is a term used to describe what happens when the body's immune system attacks itself.) The scenario goes something like this:

Inside the pancreas are approximately 100,000 cell clusters known as the **islets of Langerhans,** or **islets.** (Crossword puzzle buffs are probably very familiar with this term.) Each islet may

9

include 1,000 to 2,000 **beta cells,** which manufacture insulin and release it into the bloodstream when blood-glucose levels rise. In people with type 1 diabetes, beta cells are attacked by **antibodies,** substances created by the immune system to neutralize invading, or foreign, cells, and are slowly destroyed. Eventually, production of insulin comes to a halt because no beta cells remain.

Scientists are not quite sure what causes the body's immune system to sabotage pancreatic cells, although they have detected a genetic predisposition to this disorder. Many scientists also believe that a trigger, perhaps a virus, must be present to start the destruction. Two recent studies implicate the coxsackievirus (related to the poliovirus) as a possible trigger for type 1 diabetes. More research is needed to confirm the virus's role. We talk more about the idea of triggers in Chapter 2.

This destruction of pancreatic cells probably takes four to seven years, according to research. Unfortunately, symptoms don't arise until 80 to 90 percent of the beta cells are destroyed. Once that happens, sudden and dramatic symptoms may appear. The disease may be quickly detected and diagnosed at that point.

The symptoms of type 1 diabetes include frequent urination, constant thirst and hunger, and weight loss. Some people have fatigue, blurred vision, and recurrent skin infections. And, of course, tests will show elevated blood-sugar levels and sugar in the urine.

At present, doctors cannot prevent type 1 diabetes, nor is it something that can be avoided. But researchers are busily looking for a way to identify both the predisposing genetic factors and the viral or environmental triggers of the disease. They reason that if they can detect cell destruction early, a method of treatment known as **immunotherapy** can be used to stop the body from destroying the beta cells, thus halting the disease's progression. New areas of research are discussed in the next chapter.

TYPE 2 DIABETES

Type 2 diabetes was formally called **non-insulin-dependent diabetes, adult-onset diabetes,** and **maturity-onset diabetes** because the condition usually doesn't require insulin treatments and seldom develops in people younger than forty. However, experts are quick to point out that age is an unreliable indicator of diabetes type since a person of any age can develop type 2 diabetes. Plus, insulin is sometimes used in certain cases. As a result, the condition is now known simply as type 2 diabetes. Type 2 diabetes in children and adolescents is sometimes called **maturity-onset diabetes of the young** and given the acronym MODY.

Type 2 diabetes accounts for 90 to 95 percent of all cases of diabetes and usually shows up in middle-aged to older adults. Four out of five of these people are overweight—and in most cases, these people were overweight *before* their diabetes developed. An estimated 14.9 million people have type 2 diabetes, though one-third aren't aware of it.

To an even greater extent than with type 1, type 2 runs in families. But it's generally thought that a combination of excess weight and age triggers the genetic predisposition.

Another major difference between type 1 and type 2 diabetes is that people with type 1 diabetes must use insulin to live. As you recall, their bodies cannot produce this hormone because their beta cells have been irrevocably destroyed. Although some people with type 2 diabetes eventually become insulin dependent, most can control their blood-sugar levels through some combination of drugs, weight loss, diet, and exercise.

But the biggest difference is that people with type 2 diabetes, by controlling their disease with lifestyle changes or medical maintenance, are able to reverse the disease process so that insulin is produced and functions normally. The reversal is possible because people with type 2 diabetes still produce the hormone insulin, but it does not function properly. The malfunction is tied to being overweight. Generally, someone who is chronically obese has a high carbohydrate intake, which places a strain on the body's glucose metabolism. At the same time, obesity reduces the body's sensitivity to insulin by causing the insulin **receptors** on the cells' surfaces to stop absorbing—or to resist—insulin. Those cells (primarily muscle and fat cells) then cannot take glucose from the blood. In response to the resulting high blood sugar, beta cells in the pancreas struggle to produce more and more insulin. Eventually, this overproduction exhausts the beta cells and insulin secretion becomes inadequate.

Doctors often use the term *insulin resistance* to indicate that insulin is present but is not being used efficiently. The reason for insulin resistance is not completely understood, although scientists are striving to learn more about it. Recent research suggests that in some cases it may have to do with the way skeletal muscles store glucose for later use. For us, it's enough to know that insulin resistance plays a role in type 2 diabetes.

People with type 2 diabetes are sometimes given drugs called **oral hypoglycemic agents** to increase the secretion and effectiveness of insulin. But there's another way to achieve this goal: by cutting back on food intake and losing weight. Apparently, according to various experts, a weight loss of as little as ten to fifteen pounds can make a difference in the need for medications to control type 2 diabetes.

Although in type 2 diabetes changes in glucose levels may be mild and may be controlled with medication, there is still reason to worry about blood-sugar levels. Again, prolonged hyperglycemia—one of the disorders associated with all types of diabetes—leads to long-term complications.

Type 2 diabetes is difficult to detect for several reasons:

- The disease typically exhibits no symptoms for many years, and the onset and progression of symptoms can be slow.

- Typical symptoms are not always present.

- Symptoms are mild and may go unnoticed, which helps explain why experts estimate there are millions of people who do not know they have diabetes.

The symptoms of type 2 diabetes are similar to those of type 1 and include the following: frequent urination, increased thirst, increased hunger, prolonged and unexplained fatigue, blurred vision, numbness or tingling or burning sensations in the legs or feet, slow-healing wounds or sores, gynecological fungal infections in women, and sexual impotence in men. All too often, however, the symptoms may be very subtle, or they may imitate another disease. It may take years before symptoms manifest themselves. And in some cases, no symptoms occur at all.

Most people find out they have type 2 diabetes when a routine blood test unearths high blood-glucose levels or when they visit a doctor to be treated for symptoms of one of the complications of diabetes.

At times, a doctor may be unsure if a person has type 1 or type 2 diabetes. As we said before, there are many similarities between the symptoms of type 1 and type 2 diabetes. In the early stages of the disease, it is not always easy to determine which form someone has developed because some people experience characteristics of both. Unfortunately, there are no routine tests that can distinguish one type from another. For many doctors, the road to determining which type of diabetes a patient has is filled with trial and error. It involves trying one treatment approach and, if that doesn't work, trying another.

Your job in such a case is to become educated about diabetes and to work with health care practitioners in developing and following a treatment plan. The ultimate goal, of course, is to reach and maintain normal blood-sugar levels.

OTHER TYPES OF DIABETES

It's possible that a person may have another form of diabetes besides type 1 or type 2. Not all are truly diabetes, but they may signal that diabetes is developing. We look at four: **increased risk for diabetes, impaired glucose tolerance, secondary diabetes,** and **gestational diabetes.**

Increased Risk for Diabetes

Actually, this category is not a form of diabetes per se. But someone who is put in this group may be at increased risk of developing diabetes one day. Think of this as a warning flag, urging you to pay more attention to your health.

As described in the *Joslin Diabetes Manual*, this type of glucose abnormality includes two categories. The first refers to people with **previous abnormality of glucose tolerance** (formerly called *prediabetes*). People with this have no sign of abnormal glucose metabolism, but they experienced a period of impaired glucose tolerance or high blood sugar in the past. Women who have had gestational diabetes (which we discuss shortly) are also placed in this group.

The second category refers to people with **potential abnormality of glucose.** People who have a close relative with type 1 diabetes or people with islet-cell antibodies are considered part of this group. Doctors don't really treat people with potential abnormalities because there's really nothing to treat. Physicians should monitor the blood-sugar levels of these folks, however, in case something develops down the road.

Impaired Glucose Tolerance

Glucose tolerance is said to be impaired when blood-sugar levels are somewhat elevated but not too far beyond the normal range. Symptoms of diabetes are generally absent.

Strictly speaking, doctors don't consider impaired glucose tolerance a true form of diabetes, but instead an abnormality in glucose levels—something between normal and *overt diabetes,* as the medical profession terms it. A person who has impaired glucose tolerance may improve, with blood-sugar levels becoming normal. Or he may remain unchanged, with sugar levels steady in that gray area between normal and high. Perhaps a quarter of people with impaired glucose tolerance go on to develop diabetes, usually type 2.

It doesn't appear that impaired glucose tolerance causes severe complications of diabetes, such as kidney failure. But researchers believe that people with impaired glucose tolerance are more likely to have high blood pressure and high **cholesterol** levels—conditions long implicated in coronary heart disease. For that reason, impaired glucose tolerance needs to be treated.

Secondary Diabetes

The term *secondary diabetes* is used to describe a host of other conditions that can give rise to diabetes. In such cases, the diabetes is a secondary condition that results from another disease, medication, or chemical. Among the causes of secondary diabetes are pancreatic diseases (especially chronic pancreatitis in alcoholics), hormonal abnormalities (including ones that result from the administration of steroids), malfunctions of cells' insulin receptors, drug- or chemical-induced diabetes, and certain genetic syndromes.

In other words, drugs can induce a form of diabetes in some instances because they increase blood sugar to abnormally high levels. Certain prescription drugs, including glucocorticoids (used as anti-inflammatories), furosemide (a diuretic, used in blood-pressure control), thiazide diuretics (used in blood-pressure control), estrogen-containing products (such as oral contraceptives and hormone replacement therapy), protease inhibitors (used to treat AIDS), and beta blockers (used to treat heart disorders), may produce high blood sugar. Any diagnosis of diabetes should take into account the consumer's history of prescription drug use.

Gestational Diabetes

Gestational diabetes is any type of diabetes that first appears—or is first recognized—during pregnancy. It develops because of the distinctive hormonal environment and metabolic demands of pregnancy. Minorities and immigrants are especially at risk for gestational diabetes, reports the CDC. Native American women have the highest risk of gestational diabetes, followed by Hispanic women of Puerto Rican descent.

In 95 percent of the cases, the diabetes disappears after childbirth. For some women, however, the diabetes remains. And once a woman has had gestational diabetes, she's at risk for developing another form of diabetes (usually type 2) later in life. As just one example, Hispanic women who have gestational diabetes and impaired glucose tolerance have a 50 percent risk of developing type 2 diabetes within five years of having gestational diabetes.

An estimated 3 to 5 percent of pregnant women develop gestational diabetes. It can occur in anyone, but it seems to be more common in women over thirty, women who are overweight, and women with a family history of diabetes. The risk seems to be similar in first and subsequent pregnancies, although taking some oral contraceptives can increase the risk in women who have experienced gestational diabetes during a previous pregnancy.

Gestational diabetes symptoms are generally mild and not life threatening to the woman. However, women with gestational diabetes are more susceptible than normal to developing **toxemia,** a life-threatening condition for both mother and fetus. And gestational diabetes can pose problems for the newborn, including hypoglycemia (low blood sugar) and respiratory-distress syndrome.

Some women find they need to take insulin, but for the most part, diet and exercise can control gestational diabetes. We talk more about this form of diabetes later in the book.

Risk Factors

There is no typical, one-size-fits-all description of someone who has diabetes. All people are vulnerable to the disease throughout their lives.

Admittedly, statistics point to times of life when diabetes is more likely to occur. As one doctor describes it, "There is a gradual increase in susceptibility, with slight peaks at puberty and during pregnancy, until we reach the age of forty. Then there is a rapid jump." So it's more common to talk about

19

"susceptibility" and the risk factors associated with the disease rather than what causes it.

The top two risk factors are heredity and obesity. Diabetes can run in families, and experts term heredity the most important predisposing factor, particularly for type 1 diabetes.

Type 2 diabetes also tends to run in families. The latest scientific research suggests that in people with type 2 diabetes, several chromosomal genes that control metabolism have mutated. On their own, these defective genes do not cause diabetes, but in the presence of certain lifestyle factors, particularly obesity, a high-cholesterol diet, and physical inactivity, they may promote onset of the disease.

As we mentioned earlier, 80 to 85 percent of people with type 2 diabetes are overweight. (*Overweight* simply means weighing more than your ideal body weight, even as little as ten to twenty pounds.) True, not all overweight people have diabetes, but they could be setting themselves up for this disease ten or twenty years hence. As one expert puts it, "Events that occur in middle life (excessive weight gain, for example) can have profound clinical effects twenty years later."

Evidence also shows that the distribution of body fat affects the risk of diabetes in women. In the landmark Nurses' Health Study, which has studied more than 40,000 women for close to ten years, researchers found that women with waist circumferences of more than 36.2 inches were more likely to develop type 2 diabetes than were women with waist sizes of 36.2 inches or less. In addition, women with waist-to-hip ratios of 0.86 or more had a higher risk than women with ratios of 0.7 or less. In other words, women who carry their weight in the abdominal area are at greater risk than women whose weight is on their hips.

Data from the Nurses' Health Study also indicate that a diet high in sugar and low in fiber can significantly increase a woman's risk of type 2 diabetes. The women who consumed the most sugar and the least amount of fiber had 2.5 times the risk of those who ate little sugar and a lot of fiber.

Race is also a risk factor. In the United States, the disease is more common among African-Americans, Asians and Asian-Americans, Hispanics, and Native Americans. African-Americans are 1.7 times as likely to have type 2 diabetes than the general population. Hispanic-Americans are twice as likely. The story is worse for Native Americans, who have a prevalence of 12.2 percent, compared with 5.2 percent within the general population. In some tribes, an estimated 50 percent of the members have the disease.

Scientists stress, however, that race alone does not predict diabetes; it must be combined with another factor, such as obesity. For example, a recent National Institutes of Health study reported that being African-American isn't an independent risk factor for type 2 diabetes. The link between race and diabetes varies according to a person's weight. At 100 percent desirable weight (meaning as close as possible to ideal weight), African-Americans and Caucasians have the same risk for diabetes. But at 125 percent of desirable weight, the risk in African-Americans is 1.5 times greater than that of Caucasians. At 150 percent of desirable weight, the risk is 1.8 times greater.

Poverty is another risk factor. Two consumer surveys, conducted by the Gallup Organization in 1989 and in 1990, found a clear relationship between household income and diabetes incidence. Households with the lowest income—less than $15,000—had by far the highest incidence of the disease.

Here are a few more risk factors, some that we've already touched on in this chapter:

- Having impaired glucose tolerance.

- Having high blood pressure or high cholesterol levels (240 mg/dl or more).

- Cigarette smoking.

- Being older than age forty and having any of the preceding factors.

- In women, having a history of gestational diabetes or delivery of babies weighing more than nine pounds. There is also some evidence that babies who weigh less than average at birth—but who were not premature—may be more likely to develop diabetes later in life.

If you have any one of those risk factors, you will not necessarily get diabetes. For the most part, the presence of one risk factor does not predict diabetes, but it does suggest that it may develop. The more risk factors you have, the greater your chance of developing diabetes. According to the American Diabetes Association, the chances that a person without any risk factors will develop diabetes are low.

Diagnosing Diabetes

Primary care physicians are usually the practitioners who diagnose diabetes, mainly because they are the ones who first hear about symptoms that may indicate the condition (you can find more on doctors and diabetes in the next section).

At one time, diagnosis consisted of taste-testing the urine. If it was sweet, that was a confirmation of diabetes mellitus. Fortunately, at least for diagnosticians, things are different today. Diabetes is usually confirmed by observation of the typical signs and symptoms, as well as by tests that indicate high glucose levels in the blood and/or urine. In symptomless people, high blood sugar usually is enough for a diagnosis. On the other hand, it is possible for someone to have some glucose in the urine or mild elevations in blood-glucose levels and not have diabetes.

Because blood-glucose levels vary during the course of the day, the medical profession dictates that any tests be done while a person is **fasting.** Fasting means that the person hasn't eaten for three or more hours (before breakfast, for example). In normal adults, blood-glucose levels range between 60 and 100 milligrams per deciliter—designated as mg/dl—of blood plasma when a person is fasting. Blood-glucose numbers are slightly higher for children.

When diabetes is suspected or when a routine blood test reveals high sugar levels (above 200 mg/dl), one of two simple tests is often performed. The two tests are the **fasting plasma glucose test** and the **oral glucose-tolerance test.**

The fasting plasma glucose test is performed after a person hasn't eaten for eight to twelve hours, usually first thing in the morning. To diagnose diabetes, several of these tests are given on different days. In the past, glucose levels higher than 140 mg/dl in two successive tests confirmed diabetes. However, in June 1997, the U.S. Committee on the Diagnosis and Classification of Diabetes Mellitus lowered the cutoff to 126 mg/dl. The change is intended to diagnose diabetes, which is a progressive disease, earlier—some experts say up to five years earlier—and prevent complications. Experts estimate that the new standard will result in an additional two million Americans being classified as having diabetes.

The second test, the oral glucose-tolerance test, begins with a fasting blood sample taken after a person has eaten a high-carbohydrate diet for three days. After that sample is taken, the consumer drinks a glucose solution. Next, blood samples are taken every thirty minutes for two hours, and another sample is taken one hour later. Those blood samples show how the body handles glucose. Normally, blood levels rise after the glucose is drunk and then return to normal. In people with diabetes, blood-sugar levels don't fall that quickly. Blood-glucose levels higher than 200 mg/dl one to two hours after a meal confirm diabetes. If the blood sugar registers over 200 mg/dl after the fasting segment of this test, there's no doubt that the person has diabetes. Because the oral glucose-tolerance test is complicated and time-consuming, most practitioners rely on the fasting plasma glucose test for diagnosis.

Being Put to the Test

Along with its recommendations on the threshold for diabetes diagnosis, the U.S. Committee on the Diagnosis and Classification of Diabetes Mellitus also presented some guidelines on when individuals should be screened for the disease. According to the committee:

- People older than age forty-five should have a fasting plasma glucose test every three years. Those at high risk should be screened more often.

- Pregnant women do not need to be tested routinely if they are Caucasian, under twenty-five, of normal weight, and have no family history of diabetes.

Being diagnosed with diabetes is only the beginning—after all, the condition is a lifelong disease. A few exceptions do exist, however. For example, in cases of gestational diabetes, women may find that normal blood-sugar levels reappear. Other people with diabetes—those with type 2—may be fortunate and find that controlling their weight also controls their blood sugar.

These circumstances aside, having diabetes means making a lifelong commitment to understanding the condition and paying careful attention to diet and exercise. If you've been diagnosed with type 1 diabetes, you can find information on your condition in Chapter 2. Type 2 diabetes is discussed in Chapter 3.

Putting Together a Health Care Team

Once you've been diagnosed with diabetes, you need to find a practitioner—or practitioners—who can help you manage the disease. The good news is that most people need to look no further than a primary care doctor. Throughout the world, reports the *Joslin Diabetes Manual*, more than 90 percent of those with diabetes receive treatment from a general practitioner or internist.

You might think that a specialist would be the best choice for the treatment of a disease such as diabetes—after all, most chronic conditions are treated by specialists. However, because diabetes affects so many different parts of the body in so many different ways, a general practitioner or internist is a good

Suspect Diabetes? See Your Doctor.

To receive a diabetes diagnosis, a person should visit a physician for testing. Although there are blood-measurement kits available in the drugstore that can come in handy for those who have been diagnosed with diabetes, they shouldn't be used for self-diagnosis. These kits are used by people with diabetes to keep track of their day-to-day blood-sugar levels. As a tracking technique, **self-monitoring of blood glucose,** or **SMBG** as the medical profession calls it, plays a crucial role in managing diabetes. It gives the information needed to balance food intake, exercise, and insulin or medication. However, it's not intended to be used as a method of diagnosis.

Self-testing is an important aspect of self-care, and we talk at great length about it in Chapter 5. But for now, the major diagnostic tests are performed in a doctor's office.

choice since these doctors have experience treating the whole person, not just a particular system. Having a primary care physician treat your diabetes also ensures that you will continue to get routine care such as flu shots, cholesterol screenings, and so on.

No matter what sort of doctor you choose, it's important to have a practitioner you can rely on to coordinate your care. Getting a handle on diabetes requires not only trips to a primary care doctor but also testing at home and self-care measures such as diet and exercise programs. And no doctor is an expert in every matter, so there are times when a primary care doctor must refer a patient to a specialist. But even when your primary care doctor isn't the one providing your care, he still plays an important role in managing your treatment. A primary care doctor who can keep an eye on your total overall health and pinpoint any problems is a valuable ally in the fight against diabetes.

SEEKING SPECIALIZED CARE

But while the primary care practitioner is a key player in your treatment plan, there are times when a specialist might be called for. Specialists who might be involved with diabetes care include:

- *Endocrinologists.* These physicians specialize in treating disorders of the endocrine system, of which the pancreas is a part.

- *Neurologists.* These doctors specialize in treating nerve problems.

- *Cardiologists.* Cardiologists specialize in treating heart disease, a common complication of diabetes.

- *Ophthalmologists.* These doctors specialize in treating eye disease, also a common complication of diabetes.

Board Certification and Specialists

A specialist is a doctor who concentrates on a specific body system, age group, or disorder. In the world of medicine, prostate conditions are treated—along with other reproductive and urinary disorders in men—by a specialist known as a urologist. To become a urologist, an M.D. (doctor of medicine) or D.O. (doctor of osteopathy) must undergo two to three years of supervised specialty training, called a residency. Often a specialist also takes one or more years of additional training, called a fellowship, in a specific area of the specialty, called a subspecialty.

How can you tell if a doctor is a trained specialist? A doctor who has taken extra training in a field often chooses to become board certified. In addition to the extra training, the doctor must pass a rigorous examination administered by a specialty board, a national board of professionals in that specialty field. A doctor who passes the board examination is given the status of Diplomate. Most board-certified doctors become members of their medical specialty societies, and any doctor who meets the full requirements for membership is called a "fellow" of the society and may use the designation.

In its most basic sense, board certification indicates that a physician has completed a course of study in accordance with the established educational standards. Board certification has been

continues

called a minimum standard of excellence and nothing more. Paper certification does not produce professional excellence. On the other hand, board certification is a good sign that the person is up-to-date on the procedures, theories, and success-failure rates in the specialty. There are, however, some inferior doctors who somehow manage to become board certified and some excellent doctors without board certification.

The training requirements are similar for M.D.s and D.O.s, although they are usually certified by different boards. M.D.s are certified by one or more of the twenty-four member boards of the American Board of Medical Specialties (ABMS); D.O.s are certified by the department of certification of the American Osteopathic Association (AOA). In the case of urology, however, both osteopathic and allopathic physicians are certified by the American Board of Urology, an allopathic board, because there is no osteopathic board designated for urology.

The training programs for ABMS-recognized specialties are offered only at accredited medical schools with approved programs. There are also self-designated medical specialty boards, which are not recognized by the ABMS or the AOA and may not have the same standards and training requirements as the national boards.

You can find the names of many board-certified specialists in *The Official ABMS Directory of Board-Certified Medical Specialists* and the *American Medical Directory: Physicians in the United States,* both usually found in local libraries. The ABMS directory will also tell you where the doctor did his residency training and how long he has been practicing.

If you wish to call to verify the credentials of a specialist, you can contact the American Board of Medical Specialties at 800-776-CERT. For more information on osteopathic certification, contact the American Osteopathic Association, Department of Certification, 142 East Ontario Street, Chicago, IL 60611; 800-621-1773 or 312-280-5845.

Not every specialist who may be involved in your care is a medical doctor. A podiatrist, a health care professional who specializes in foot care, may be enlisted to handle a foot ulcer or similar problem. A dietitian, who specializes in nutrition, may be called upon to design a diet that will suit your needs. A physical therapist or personal trainer may help put together an exercise program that will help lower blood sugar levels.

PARTICIPATING IN YOUR CARE

All of the people involved in your treatment make up your diabetes care team. But don't forget that you are a member of that team as well. Diabetes is an ongoing, complicated disease that requires regular trips to your physician and self-care and monitoring at home. Don't visit your doctor just when you're having a problem—make an effort to get long-term, ongoing care.

How often do you need to visit your doctor? The answer to that question is a function of many factors. According to the American Diabetes Association, four visits a years is the norm for people who use insulin or who have unstable blood-sugar levels. People with well-controlled diabetes should see their doctors two to four times a year. Complications, illness, or changes in a treatment plan may make more visits necessary.

CHOOSING A PHYSICIAN

Choosing a doctor is always a personal matter. You want someone who will listen to your opinions and treat you with respect—in short, someone who will treat you as an equal partner in health care. Whether you choose someone who specializes in diabetes care or someone whose treatment methods lean away from the medical mainstream, this is a decision that only you can make. However, it's important that your practitioner strive to keep you as healthy as possible.

If you don't have a physician and hope to get one, begin your search by getting a few good recommendations from family members, friends, and neighbors. Don't overlook your primary care provider, either. Other sources to consider are:

- Physician referral services operated by the local medical society (usually county-based) and local hospitals. However, such services will refer only those practitioners who are members and will not comment on the ability of providers other than to perhaps mention their board certifications.

- The company personnel office. Companies sometimes use certain practitioners for employment physicals and disability claims.

- Health insurance companies, which can sometimes be helpful when you require a specialist for a second opinion.

- Listings in the telephone directory. Practitioners' names are usually arranged according to practice or specialty, but remember that doctors can practice in any specialty area they choose, whether or not they have had any advanced training. Look for board certification.

- Nurses or other medical professionals.

- Senior centers. Some have lists of practitioners either affiliated with or recommended by the center.

Once you've found a few practitioners in your area in which you are interested, the next step is a face-to-face meeting. Call the office for an appointment and mention that you would be a new patient; then ask to arrange a get-acquainted visit, a fifteen-minute meeting during which you can ask questions and find out a little more about the practitioner. Be aware that some practitioners charge for these appointments.

During the visit, evaluate the office and staff. Ask a receptionist about the procedures for making appointments, telephoning the practitioner, getting prescription refills, and obtaining copies of medical records.

Because the meeting with the practitioner is short, have your questions ready. You will want to know the practitioner's medical degree, board certification, and hospital affiliations. Ask about fees and payment plans.

This is also an opportunity to discover the philosophy of the practitioner, the attitude toward alternative therapies, and whether the patient is seen as a full partner in health care. Also notice the attitude of the practitioner. Are your questions heard and answered in a forthright manner? You will also want to consider:

- Is the practice solo or group?

- If group, are the practitioners the same specialty?

- If group, are the practitioners different specialties?

- Does this practitioner publish or make available a list of fees and current charges?

- Does the office appear neat and clean? Are there current magazines?

- Is your insurance coverage accepted? Will the office file all insurance claims?

- Does the staff maintain a professional, friendly attitude?

- Was your appointment kept on time?

CREATING A TREATMENT PLAN

Once you have enlisted the help of a physician, you need to work with that doctor to create a treatment plan that will spell out how you will try to meet the main goal of diabetes treatment: keeping blood-sugar levels as close to normal as possible.

According to the American Diabetes Association, a complete diabetes care plan includes:

- A list of long-term and short-term goals.

- A list of medications prescribed to control diabetes.

- Advice from a dietitian on diet therapy.

- Educational sessions on how to monitor blood-sugar and urine ketone levels and how to treat reactions to low blood-sugar levels.

- A plan for seeing a dentist, eye doctor, foot doctor, or other specialists, if necessary.

- A birth control or pregnancy plan for women.

Everyone's care plan is different and must be designed specifically with that person's needs in mind. In the following chapters, you can find information on some of the specifics of diabetes. Chapter 2 presents the details about type 1 diabetes and the use of insulin, so if you're facing type 1—or have type 2 diabetes and use insulin—this is the place to start. Those with type 2 diabetes can find the information they need in Chapter 3, which talks about the condition and the medications available to keep it in check. Chapter 4 discusses some of the complications of both type 1 and type 2 diabetes—that is, some of the problems that may arise if they are not adequately controlled. In Chapter 5, you can find information about self-care and your own very important role in treatment.

CHAPTER TWO

Type 1 Diabetes and the Importance of Insulin

IF YOU OR SOMEONE YOU LOVE HAS BEEN DIAGNOSED WITH TYPE 1 diabetes, you'll soon find out that managing the condition depends largely on one thing in the long run: insulin. As was explained in Chapter 1, type 1 diabetes was known once as insulin-dependent diabetes because, in general, people with type 1 diabetes lose the ability to manufacture the hormone insulin. Thus, they need to receive insulin, most frequently in the form of injections, to regulate the way their bodies use food for energy.

In this chapter, we talk about the different types of insulin available, the factors that will determine your insulin regimen, and the ways in which insulin can be administered. We also touch on some advanced treatments for type 1 diabetes, such as pancreatic transplants, as well as new ways in which researchers are working to prevent the disease.

If you're facing type 2 diabetes, don't automatically skip to the next chapter. Most people with type 2 diabetes (once called non-insulin-dependent diabetes) are able to control their blood-sugar levels through some combination of drugs, weight loss, diet, and exercise. However, some become dependent on insulin—sometimes intermittently, sometimes for life. In those cases, much of what we talk about in this chapter applies to them as well.

How Does Insulin Work?

Insulin injections cannot cure diabetes. Insulin injections merely compensate for the hormone's absence from the body. They modify the symptoms of the disease, but they don't treat the cause.

Insulin controls diabetes that cannot be controlled by diet alone, but it's not a replacement for diet either. If people with diabetes are not careful about what and how much they eat, they will not be able to control their blood-sugar levels, regardless of insulin intake.

Although this chapter focuses on the role of insulin and how people use it, the fact is that people with type 1 diabetes need both insulin injections and regimented diets to live. Diet is such an important issue for all people with diabetes that we've devoted the lion's share of Chapter 5 to that topic.

The words "discipline" and "regimented" are often associated with diabetes. Most people with insulin-dependent diabetes lead fairly structured lives. Insulin intake, meals, and exercise are carefully scheduled and regulated. All this structure is necessary to keep blood sugar in a normal range, called **normoglycemia** or **euglycemia.**

Controlling blood sugar is like walking a tightrope between having too much and too little sugar in the blood. Too much sugar (hyperglycemia) over the years leads to the life-threatening ailments discussed in Chapter 1. Too little sugar (hypoglycemia) causes irritability, fainting, or even death. Eating the right foods in the right amounts and maintaining the proper amount of insulin in the bloodstream are all essential to keeping your footing.

Types of Insulin

There are several kinds, or **species,** of insulin, each with a different source. **Beef-derived insulin** is obtained from beef pancreases; **pork-derived insulin** comes from pork pancreases. **Human insulin,** a drug chemically identical to the insulin normally produced by the body, is manufactured in one of two ways: either by using DNA technology or by chemical modification of pork insulin. The human insulins are known as **synthetic** and **semi-synthetic,** respectively.

Each species of insulin comes in different forms, each of which acts in a different way. Traditionally, these forms are short-acting, intermediate-acting, and long-acting.

Short-acting insulins are also called **regular** and **semilente** insulins. (Short-acting insulins are sometimes referred to as fast-acting insulins; the word *fast* refers to the speed with which the insulin begins to lower blood-sugar levels.) Most short-acting insulins begin acting in thirty to forty-five minutes, reach their peak effectiveness in one to three hours, and work for a duration of five to eight hours.

One short-acting insulin, called lispro—approved in 1996 by the U.S. Food and Drug Administration (FDA)—works even more quickly and has a shorter duration. A genetically reengineered form of short-acting, or regular, human insulin, lispro takes effect within ten minutes, peaks in forty-five minutes to one hour, and lasts three hours.

Intermediate-acting insulins come in two forms: **lente** and **NPH.** Preparations with a predetermined proportion of NPH mixed with regular insulin, such as 70 percent NPH to 30 percent regular, are considered intermediate-acting insulins. These begin acting in about one and one-half hours, reach their peak in four to fourteen hours, and work for eighteen to twenty-four hours.

Long-acting insulins include **PZI** (short for prolamine zinc insulin) and **ultralente.** These begin to take effect in four to twelve hours, peak at twelve to twenty-four hours after injection, and last from twenty to thirty-six hours.

Most people with type 1 diabetes use several forms of insulin to control their conditions. One common approach is to use one form in the morning and another form later in the day. Other people mix insulin forms in the same syringe because they and their doctors have found that mixtures of short-acting with intermediate- or long-acting insulins do a better job of keeping blood-sugar levels normal than does use of a single insulin alone. The most commonly used insulins today are regular, semilente, NPH, lente, and ultralente.

Because different types of insulin have different pharmacological properties, one form may be preferred over another. According to a report in the journal *Diabetes Care,* human insulin is recommended for women who are pregnant or considering pregnancy, for people who are allergic to animal-derived insulins, for people who are just beginning insulin therapy, and for those who must use insulin only intermittently. In fact, most people today are started on human insulin unless they need the long-acting variety, which only comes in beef- or pork-derived forms.

Onset and Absorbency of Insulin

Aside from their origins and forms, there are other differences in insulins. Insulins vary in three important ways: how quickly the insulin takes effect (doctors use the words **onset** and **absorbency**

Insulin Allergies

It is true that a person with diabetes can be allergic to certain types of insulin. In particular, beef- and pork-derived insulins, the oldest members of the insulin family, can cause allergic reactions around the spot where the insulin was injected (known as the **injection site**).

Reactions can range in intensity from a small, red, or itchy area to a widespread skin rash, stomach upset, and even difficult breathing. Obviously, it's not something people want to endure. People who have an allergy to one form of insulin should switch to another.

Today, many animal insulins have been purified, meaning they are manufactured with fewer impurities, so allergies are less common. The purest insulins are the human insulins, made through the high-tech processes we mentioned earlier. (Just for the record, today's animal insulins are 99.99 percent pure; human insulins are 99.999 percent pure!) Since the semisynthetic and synthetic human insulins are chemically identical to the body's own insulin, they do not cause allergic reactions. More and more people with diabetes are using human insulins—which, not surprisingly, are more expensive than the older beef- or pork-derived insulins.

when talking about this), the intensity of effect or activity it creates (**degree**), and how long the effect lasts (**duration**). For example, human insulins have a more rapid onset and shorter duration of activity than pork insulins. Beef insulins have the slowest onset and longest duration of activity.

All three of these factors are important, but people with diabetes are often most concerned with onset and absorbency. As we noted, onset and absorbency have to do with when the insulin takes effect. People with diabetes need to know when the insulin kicks in because their meals are planned around the presence of an appropriate insulin boost. Without that insulin, people who are insulin dependent can't absorb and convert carbohydrates and sugars into energy.

It's always a challenge to predict accurately how quickly insulin will take effect. A person with diabetes can't be sure insulin will absorb at the same rate after each injection. In fact, absorption time differs an average of 25 percent! In other words, many factors influence how well and how quickly insulin is absorbed.

The foremost factor is the insulin itself. Absorbency differs from manufacturer to manufacturer, even within the same form of insulin. That's why insulin users generally stick to the same form (short-, intermediate-, or long-acting), the same species (human, beef, or pork), and the same brand (manufacturer) as long as possible. However, from time to time, you and your doctor may find that a change in species or brand of insulin may be necessary to keep pace with the current path of your disease.

Another important factor—and one that the individual has control over—is the injection site. Insulin is absorbed at different speeds, depending on where it is injected. Injection in the abdomen has the fastest rate of absorption, followed by the arms, thighs, and buttocks. Depending upon the person, absorption time for the abdomen might be thirty minutes, while in the thigh it might be forty-five minutes. Exercising the arm or leg after injection increases the speed of absorption. In addition, insulin works faster when it's injected in lean rather than fat areas, which is why injection into the buttocks offers the slowest absorption rate of all sites.

Whether fast absorption or slow absorption is better is entirely up to you and your meal plan. As long as you know the anticipated result, you can calculate when and where to inject your insulin.

It's a complicated proposition, keeping up with all the factors. And there are more to deal with. Injection techniques, exercise, stress, traveling, hormonal changes (such as menstruation or puberty), and even a person's individual metabolism affect insulin's onset, degree, and duration and, as a result, a person's blood-sugar levels.

Dosage and Timing

The size of a dose of insulin matters, too. As a rule, dosage varies from person to person. Insulin comes in concentrations

At the Pharmacy

When you're purchasing insulin, there are certain things you should look for. The most important step is to double-check the bottles to be sure you are getting the correct type, strength, and brand. This is particularly important if you purchase premixed insulins because they can be prepared in all sorts of combinations.

Pharmacists are not supposed to change your insulin preparations in any way without your doctor's approval—or without informing you—but mix-ups can happen. When you go shopping for insulin, take along an empty bottle that has your information on it so that you can confirm that your new prescription is the same. Or keep a copy of a label in your wallet to help you verify that you have the right stuff.

Finally, check the expiration date before you leave the store. Will you be able to use all the insulin before it expires? If not, ask for another bottle with a different shelf date.

of 40, 100, or 500 units per milliliter (written as U-40, U-100, and U-500). Most people use U-100. The appropriate dose depends on the way an individual's body responds to planned diet and exercise regimens. Virtually all type 1 and many type 2 patients need two or more injections daily to prevent blood-sugar levels from getting too low during the day while maintaining blood-sugar levels through the night.

And along with everything else to contend with, people must plan around specific times of the day for injections. The best time for an injection depends on blood-sugar levels, food consumption, exercise, and forms of insulin used.

Generally, doctors recommend an interval of thirty minutes between the injection of short-acting insulin and eating a meal. They discourage people from eating within a few minutes after (or before) injecting short-acting insulin because that substantially reduces the insulin's ability to prevent a rapid rise in blood sugar and, thus, increases the risk of hypoglycemia a few hours later. The consumer and the health care practitioner can set up guidelines for the suggested interval between insulin injection and mealtime based on factors such as blood-sugar levels, site of injection, and anticipated activity during the interval.

This is a lot of information to have to juggle at one time, but the process can be made easier. For one thing, the physician should set up a daily treatment plan that spells out elements such as dosage, insulin concentration, type of syringe, and timing of injections.

The physician should also prepare an **algorithm** for a diabetic patient—a simple mathematical chart that can serve as a guide for determining how many units of insulin to take and when to take them, depending upon blood-sugar level. There's one hitch to using an algorithm, however: The person must regularly test blood-glucose levels.

This regular testing is called self-monitoring of blood glucose, or SMBG. We mentioned it briefly in Chapter 1, and we discuss it in depth in Chapter 5. Basically, it's a way of monitoring blood-sugar fluctuations throughout the day so that the person with diabetes can do a better job of reaching target blood-sugar levels.

To do self-monitoring, a person with diabetes uses a blood-glucose meter (available at most corner drugstores) to measure the blood-sugar level in a drop of blood. The test takes forty-five seconds to two minutes to give results. With the blood-glucose measurement literally in hand, the person then looks at the algorithm for guidance on how many units of insulin to inject.

The algorithm is a handy tool, but because each algorithm varies from person to person, no one can follow anyone else's. An algorithm also needs constant reevaluation and occasional updating because diabetes is one disease that doesn't stay still.

Insulin Therapies: Standard Therapy vs. Tight Control

How often you use insulin depends upon what blood-sugar levels you and your doctor are trying to maintain.

Basically, there are two types of insulin therapy. The first is known as the **standard,** or **conventional, therapy.** Standard diabetes treatment generally entails two insulin shots a day. The **mixed-split regimen** (mixtures of intermediate-acting and short-acting insulin given before breakfast and dinner) is the most commonly used conventional regimen. Along with this comes SMBG one or two times a day.

The second, newer approach is called **tight control,** or **intensive therapy.** According to the definition created by researchers working in the Diabetes Control and Complications Trial, a large ten-year study concluded in 1993, intensive therapy is one in which people with type 1 diabetes strive to maintain near-normal blood-sugar levels either by going on an **insulin pump** (we talk about this shortly) or by taking three or more insulin injections daily and performing at least four self-administered tests of blood-glucose levels per day.

The advantage of standard treatment is that it's a fairly easy regimen to follow. The drawback is that it's fairly inflexible. Once you take your morning insulin, for instance, you can't change the time of your meals or their size —at least not without throwing blood-sugar levels out of whack. It's difficult to make spur-of-the-moment changes— not to mention hold down a job that requires travel or swing shifts—and still keep blood sugar under control.

Tight control was developed to help remedy some of the drawbacks of standard treatment and to make the diabetes treatment program more responsive to a person's lifestyle, rather than change a person's lifestyle to fit his treatment program. With the technique of tight control, people with diabetes take more frequent, smaller injections of insulin each day. As a result, they have more flexibility in the timing of meals and exercise. Many doctors believe that when a patient has more flexibility, he is more likely to follow a treatment approach.

The second goal of tight-control therapy is also the one that carries the most weight with many in the medical profession: People who can maintain close-to-normal blood-sugar levels can dramatically slow down progression of the disease. What do we mean by dramatic? According to the findings of the Diabetes Control and Complications Trial and of a smaller study in Sweden, people with type 1 diabetes may reduce *by 50 to 70 percent* their risk of developing eye problems, nerve problems, kidney disease, and other diabetic complications later in life.

In addition, many people feel physically better with a tight-control regimen, and they like the sense of empowerment they gain from being able to keep their blood sugar in a narrow range. Some experts recommend tight control to adolescents because it's so successful in staving off long-term complications.

With those results, it sounds as if everyone with diabetes should go on intensive, or tight-control, therapy. However, many people with diabetes don't want to devote that much effort to managing their disease. They are used to the standard regimen of two shots a day, and they don't want (or need) to invest the time and energy in a demanding routine of frequent injections and blood tests day after day after day. And for someone who has just been diagnosed with diabetes, the standard regimen may be a better introduction to self-care basics because the routine is simpler.

But the big concern and the source of some controversy with tight control is that blood-sugar levels can get too low, leading to hypoglycemia. Also known as an **insulin reaction** or a low-blood-sugar attack, hypoglycemia is caused by too much insulin in the bloodstream. As we mentioned in Chapter 1, early symptoms of hypoglycemia include trembling, hunger, weakness, and irritability. If blood glucose drops too low, a person may pass out, go into a coma, and eventually die.

There are several factors that can provoke hypoglycemia:

- Delaying or skipping a meal.

- Not eating enough carbohydrates in a meal.

- Suddenly increasing exercise.

- Suddenly eating a sugary meal when on a low-calorie, low-carbohydrate diet.

- Taking too much insulin.

We talk more about hypoglycemia and how to treat it in Chapter 4. But for now, it's enough to say that it's a situation people want to avoid.

Exactly how much does tight control have to do with hypoglycemia? The Diabetes Control and Complications Trial found that people following an intensive therapy of tight control experienced 3.3 times more instances of severe hypoglycemia— in other words, reactions so intense that they required the assistance of another person to recover. Yet the trial also found that although adults on tight control may have more hypoglycemic episodes, those episodes didn't cause attention, memory, learning, or motor-skills problems or a perceived drop in the quality of life. Studies referenced in the *Wall Street Journal,* however, estimated that between 4 and 13 percent of the deaths of people with type 1 diabetes are caused by hypoglycemia-related accidents. How much of this is related to a regimen of tight control is unknown.

Despite these drawbacks, doctors continue to support tight control. Many well-known physicians (including Gordon Weir, M.D., former medical director of the Joslin Diabetes Center in Falmouth, Massachusetts) stand squarely behind tight control, despite the likelihood of hypoglycemia. Proponents argue that patients on tight control can achieve admirably low and stable blood-sugar levels. They point to the 1993 statistics showing that compared with standard therapy, tight control can reduce the risk of eye disease by 76 percent, nerve damage by 60 percent, and kidney damage by 50 percent. No one disputes the significance of these benefits. For this reason, the Diabetes Control and Complications Trial concluded that tight control should be standard care.

It should also be noted that preventing hypoglycemia is generally simple—as we'll see in Chapter 5. Ultimately, too, proponents point to long-term cost savings using tight-control, or intensive, therapy. Diabetes treatment currently costs this nation close to $92 billion a year in health care and lost productivity. While intensive therapy doubles the annual cost of treatment for a person with diabetes, that is ultimately much less expensive than treating the complications of the disease.

As a precaution, be sure to choose a physician who understands this type of therapy. Both primary care practitioners and specialists may have experience. To find out whether your own doctor has experience, simply ask about qualifications. Has the doctor often prescribed tight-control therapy? How many patients does the doctor have who are on the program? Has the doctor attended any seminars or continuing education programs on tight control? If your doctor seems uncertain about how to use the therapy effectively, get a second opinion about your treatment plan.

Injecting Insulin

When insulin is prescribed, your practitioner or another health professional will discuss with you the fine points of preparing your injection and administering it. If you have any questions or are confused about how to inject the medication, be sure to contact your practitioner right away.

Look Out!

A number of additional factors, including drug interactions and your health, can affect how your insulin takes effect. As a smart consumer, you should discuss potential interactions anytime you take more than one medication, be it a prescription drug or an over-the-counter preparation. Public Citizen's *Health Letter* warns that even aspirin, cold remedies, antacids, laxatives, and smoking deterrents (such as nicotine patches) may affect the way insulin works and may mean that your dose of insulin should be adjusted. When in doubt about interactions, ask. When not in doubt, double-check!

And you should definitely not stop taking insulin if you become sick. Illness changes the effect of insulin. In some cases, you may be able to reduce your insulin dose, but most of the time you'll need to take more insulin. Call your doctor for instructions on adjusting your treatment. Blood sugar can skyrocket during an illness, especially if you have a cold, flu, infection, or injury.

Most practitioners recommend that you keep your insulin bottle at room temperature, because cold insulin can be painful when injected and may not be absorbed as well. Insulin remains stable—in other words, usable and effective—up to three months without refrigeration.

A few practitioners, however, recommend that you refrigerate the bottle you're currently using. Their advice is based on evidence that unrefrigerated insulin sometimes loses potency after the bottle has been in use for more than thirty days. The loss in potency is slight, which is why most doctors don't believe that refrigeration is necessary.

All the experts do agree on two things: People with diabetes should have on hand a spare bottle of each type of insulin used, and vials of insulin not in use should be refrigerated. But don't freeze them, and be sure to keep them away from heat and direct sunlight.

There are a few obvious signs that insulin has lost its potency. A "yes" answer to any one question signals a loss in potency:

- The expiration date has passed. If so, open a new bottle.

- The bottle has been open and unrefrigerated for more than three months. If you store insulin at room temperature, write the date on the bottle when you open it.

- The insulin looks different. Inspect insulin before you use it. Has it changed in color or clarity? (In general, short-acting insulin is clear and other insulins are uniformly cloudy.) Is there a sediment on the bottom of the bottle? Have small lumps or clumps formed?

Once you've checked the insulin and it appears fine, you can load the syringe.

Next, you need to choose an injection site. Rotating sites ensures that you're not injecting insulin into the same spot each time and helps prevent the skin from becoming thickened or scarred (which delays absorption). Most people inject insulin into the thighs, but the upper arms and abdomen are also options (as we mentioned before, the choice of injection site can affect the rate at which the insulin is absorbed, so ask your doctor). Within each area, injection sites should be changed daily. For example, a person would inject in a straight line further down the thigh each day, then begin a second or third column, then switch to the other thigh, then the abdomen, and so on.

Once the site is chosen, the injection is administered. Again, talk with your health care provider about the technique; injection methods are best demonstrated one-on-one. In addition, reread the instruction sheet that you should have received when you purchased your insulin and syringes. Here are a few basics:

- Clean your hands and the injection site before each injection. Wipe the top of the insulin vial with 70 percent isopropyl alcohol. For all insulin preparations except short-acting ones, the vial should be gently rolled in the palms of the hands to resuspend the insulin. Don't shake it—that might cause a loss of potency. After the insulin is drawn into a syringe, check the insulin for air bubbles. Give the upright syringe one or two quick flicks with the forefinger to encourage air bubbles to escape. Bubbles decrease the size of the dose.

- Ask for help if you're not feeling confident about using a syringe; improper cleansing or injection technique may lead to an infection.

Syringes can be reused. If you have glass syringes, you must keep them clean and sterilize them periodically. Reusable syringes and needles can be stored in alcohol between injections and should be boiled once a week. As for reusing disposable syringes—that's another issue debated in the medical world. Disposable syringes and needles are made for one use. Manufacturers won't guarantee the sterility of reused syringes. But since the cost of disposable syringes and needles really adds up over the course of a year, many people prefer to reuse a syringe until its needle becomes dull.

United States Pharmacopeia medical panels do not recommend reusing syringes and needles, according to an article in *Health Letter*. But the American Diabetes Association acknowledges that syringe reuse appears both safe and practical for many people with diabetes. The reason, they say, is that most insulin preparations contain additives that inhibit the growth of bacteria commonly found on the skin.

According to the American Diabetes Association, do not reuse a disposable syringe under any of the following conditions:

- Someone else used it.

- The needle is dull or bent.

- The needle came into contact with any surface other than your skin.

- You forgot to recap the needle.

- You have an infection or open wounds on your hands.

- The skin around the injection site is red or infected.

- You are ill or your resistance to infection is low.

There is a lot published nowadays about the risk of AIDS associated with sharing needles. AIDS is not going to pose a problem if you are the only person who uses the syringe. To repeat what we've said above: You should not reuse a syringe if someone else has used it. Never share one! To do so is foolhardy at best.

If you plan on reusing syringes, you should have excellent personal hygiene, good eyesight, and the hand-eye coordination necessary to recap the needle without accidentally sticking yourself. Otherwise, you put yourself at risk of infection. Make it a habit to periodically inspect the skin around the injection site. If you see unusual redness or signs of infection, discard the syringe and consult your doctor to see if you have an infection.

Some doctors recommend that you wipe the needle with alcohol after each use. Others argue that using alcohol to cleanse the needle offers no clear benefit; they add that alcohol may remove the needle's silicon coating and, thus, make injection more painful.

And how much does insulin therapy cost? According to a study in *Diabetes Spectrum*, the annual cost of standard insulin treatment for a person with type 1 diabetes is, on average, around $1,100. For tight-control therapy, the cost is about $3,300. Most of these expenses are reimbursed by insurers.

Beyond Needles: Alternatives to Injection

Many people with diabetes accept syringes as part of their self-care, while others have difficulty overcoming their distaste of needles. The good news is that a host of alternative devices for delivering insulin are available or in development. Let's look at some of them.

INSULIN PUMPS

Insulin pumps—or infusion pumps, as they are more precisely called—are small battery-operated devices that pump insulin into the body at specified intervals. They include a small mechanical motor; a display window for reading measurements; a battery; a small supply of insulin (enough for several days); and a small tube, or **catheter,** connected to a needle through which the insulin flows under the skin.

Worn on a belt or strapped to the body, pumps release insulin through the catheter at frequent, prescheduled times. Today's pumps are programmed to deliver less insulin during the period when blood sugar is likely to be down (usually the middle of the night) and more insulin for those times that blood sugar tends to rise (usually early in the morning, which is called the **"dawn phenomenon"**). Every few days, the catheter is removed and the needle reinserted at a different site (to prevent scarring and thickening of the skin), the pump's battery is changed, and the pump's supply of insulin is replenished.

In medical lingo, therapy with an infusion pump is called **continuous subcutaneous insulin infusion (CSII).** Although pumps are now available at neighborhood doctors' offices, some experts insist that consumers should have the pumps hooked up only at medical facilities with a skilled professional team (including a physician experienced in CSII therapy) capable of providing continuous care in case problems develop. People using a pump should visit their practitioner regularly for evaluation; the frequency of such visits varies according to the person's needs.

Aside from avoiding syringes, there are other advantages to using an insulin pump. In some patients, pumps and CSII therapy provide the same kind of improvement in blood-sugar control as multiple insulin injections (the "tight control" we spoke about earlier). And insulin pumps, like frequent injections, provide more flexibility in mealtimes. The user can also program in an extra burst of insulin if needed.

Some doctors recommend CSII only when three or four daily injections fail to control blood sugar. But other doctors see it as a matter of consumer choice. The best candidates for therapy are people who are strongly motivated to improve their sugar levels and who have the discipline to regularly monitor their blood-sugar levels through self-testing.

Like any therapy based on a mechanical device, pump therapy can pose a few potential complications, and anyone who uses an infusion pump needs to be aware of them. For instance, undetected interruptions in insulin delivery may result in episodes of extremely high blood sugar, which is why frequent blood-sugar tests are essential. Infections and inflammation at the site where the needle is inserted under the skin are other potential complications, but they can be minimized by careful hygiene and by changing the needle site frequently.

And then there's the issue of appearance, which is more important to some people than others. Although infusion pumps come in many sizes, most of them are about the size of a paging beeper. People using the pump should not be off the pump for more than one hour without the use of additional insulin, although the pump can be disconnected briefly to allow for bathing, sexual activity, exercise, and the like. The pump is worn during sleep.

IMPLANTABLE PUMPS

The pumps are becoming smaller and more inconspicuous every year. But for the most inconspicuous pump of all, the award goes to the newest development in pump therapy: the **implantable pump,** also known as the **closed-loop pump.** This small device, which is surgically inserted under the skin, is still being studied and is not yet available to the average medical consumer.

The implantable pump, about the size of a hockey puck, is a complete unit inserted within the body, often in the abdominal area. Insertion is done during a thirty- to ninety-minute procedure performed using either local or general anesthesia. In theory, a pump closely imitates the insulin actions of the pancreas. There are no long tubes or view windows because these little computerized pumps decide how much insulin is needed and then automatically release it. About every one to three months, the pumps need to be refilled. This is done through a short procedure in which a needle is inserted through the skin into the pump and its reservoir is refilled with insulin via a syringe.

The idea is that implantable insulin-delivery pumps provide even more precise insulin delivery because they are not affected by skin temperature, exercise, and other variables that affect absorption of insulin injected by syringe.

As a way of helping diabetic people achieve and maintain normal blood-sugar levels, implantable pumps seem to be developing a good track record. Research on one model found that up to 50 percent of people with type 1 diabetes brought their blood-sugar levels to normal—pretty good results for insulin-dependent diabetes. And another clinical trial of a programmable implantable medication system (PIMS) reported no surgical or skin complications, severe episodes of low blood sugar, or instances of extremely high (over 1,000 mg/dl) blood sugar.

There have been some problems with implants, but most have been resolved. According to an article in the *New England Journal of Medicine,* implanted pumps had plenty of problems in studies during the early 1980s. Insulin tended to collect within the pump or catheter, batteries had a short life, and mechanical failures were frequent. Most of those problems seem to have disappeared in the implanted pumps of the 1990s. Catheter blockages are still the most common complication, but they can be overcome by changing the catheter under local anesthetic.

One drawback to the pump may be cost. Although the pumps are not yet available to the public, the anticipated price for a pump is estimated to be $10,000 to $15,000—not including the cost of sugery, which could amount to another $2,000 to $5,000. Pump refills and doctors' visits are another expense, and if complications occur, additional surgery or medical treatment may need to be paid for. It is unlikely that insurance companies will cover the expense since less costly alternatives to the pump are available.

And as good as they sound, implanted pumps have a rather short life span—fifteen to thirty months, according to several pilot studies. The pump then must be surgically removed and replaced with another.

JET INJECTORS

As the name implies, jet injectors use pressure to shoot insulin into the skin with jetlike speed. An injector is used just as a syringe would be. However, injectors are a bit larger than a syringe and have no needles. Thus, they are particularly useful devices for adults who are so frightened by needles that they don't take insulin as often as directed.

Not exactly new, jet injection was first proposed for use with insulin in the 1950s. Today's injectors appear to be mechanically reliable and accurate. Compared with syringe injection, insulin absorption and distribution differ when administered by jet injection. In general, jet-injected insulin decreases blood-sugar levels more than an equal amount of insulin administered by syringe does—meaning that less jet-injected insulin is needed to do the job.

Of course, there are drawbacks to jet injectors. Some people complain that jet injectors are cumbersome to sterilize, while others point out that jet injection is not necessarily less painful than a needle. A few doctors still have concerns about the consistency of the delivered insulin dose, but on the whole, jet injectors have an established place among the ranks of insulin-delivery devices.

INSULIN PENS

Like syringes, insulin pens use needles to inject insulin. But instead of having to handle vials of insulin, the user simply pops in a cartridge of insulin, indicates the appropriate number of units of insulin, and shoots the insulin in.

As the name suggests, these devices are shaped like pens. Disposable needles attach at one end. Insulin pens are popular with people who take multiple daily injections of insulin, as in the intensive, or tight-control, regimen.

ON THE HORIZON

Down the road, researchers are talking about developing an insulin pill, and one pharmacologist at Texas A & M College of Medicine predicts that the day is coming when people may take insulin through an eyedropper.

The most promising innovation to date is an inhaled form of regular insulin. In June 1998, researchers from the University of Miami announced successful clinical trials of inhaled insulin at the American Diabetes Association's Annual Scientific Sessions. The insulin is delivered through a device similar to an asthma inhaler. It sends a dose of powdered insulin through the mouth and directly into the lungs where it can easily be absorbed into the bloodstream. Trials of the device, which is being developed by Pfizer, Inc., are continuing;

The Issue of Cost

None of the high-tech devices we've been talking about here is inexpensive. But if they are what you need to take control—and if they help you follow your treatment regimen—then you may decide they are worth the price.

Insulin pumps are expensive, costing $3,000 to $5,000. Supplies to use them can run another $3,600 a year. Jet injectors and insulin pens are less expensive than infusion pumps, for obvious reasons. Even so, depending upon how many syringes you use in a year, experts estimate that it may take two to five years to recoup the cost of something like a jet injector. (As you recall, standard insulin therapy with syringes costs about $1,100 a year, while tight-control therapy runs about $3,300.)

Insurance coverage of these devices varies from company to company, although more plans are beginning to cover the new devices when prescribed by a physician.

however, approval from FDA may take another three to five years.

The Fight Against Diabetes

Clearly, treatment and maintenance programs to help limit the implications of diabetes are valuable. But what about preventing diabetes in the first place? What about finding a cure?

PREVENTING DIABETES

Both diabetes triggers—factors that spark diabetes onset—and diabetes markers—genetic "signposts"—are the focus of current research into diabetes prevention. The idea is that one day doctors can find those people who will get diabetes and can stop the disease before it starts.

Triggers are external environmental factors, such as exposure to a virus, exposure to certain chemicals, or nutritional habits, that trigger an inherited, or genetic, predisposition to diabetes. Scientists think many different triggers may be responsible for 70 to 95 percent of type 1 cases.

As research progresses, doctors are finding these triggers. One study, reported in the *New England Journal of Medicine,* points to cow's milk in infants as an environmental trigger of type 1 diabetes. The article notes, "This study strongly suggests that antibodies to albumin in cow's milk also attack the child's own pancreatic beta cells; thus an immunologic reaction to cow's milk may precipitate diabetes in susceptible children." Based on those findings, the American Academy of Pediatrics recommends that parents *do not* give whole cow's milk to infants under one year of age. In addition, some experts believe that breast-fed infants may be protected against the risk of type 1 diabetes later in life.

Other triggers are also under investigation. As mentioned in Chapter 1, researchers are exploring initial reports that implicate coxsackieviruses (related to the poliovirus) as possible triggers for type 1 diabetes. Another theory is that vaccines given to young children might cause inflammation of the islet cells in the pancreas and trigger diabetes. Research is underway to determine if there is any connection between immunization and diabetes.

Some advances are also taking place in the area of identifying genetic markers—those genetic indications that a person may develop diabetes. For example, one marker appears to be changes in the way the pancreas secretes insulin. Scientists can use special blood tests to identify, with near certainty among first-degree relatives of people with type 1 diabetes, those who will develop diabetes. These assays, as the tests are called, identify individuals with insulin or islet-cell antibodies.

More research is under way. According to *The Joslin Diabetes Manual,* other researchers have located two **antigens** (proteins or enzymes capable of stimulating action in the immune system) that serve as markers. These antigens, known as HLA-B8 and HLA-B15, are attacked by the antibodies and white blood cells that make up part of the body's immune system. HLA-B8 and HLA-B15 are more common in people with type 1 diabetes than in people without diabetes.

This information is valuable to researchers. Because scientists have the ability to predict the development of type 1 diabetes in some people, investigators have begun to halt or even prevent beta-cell destruction in such individuals.

This might even mean preventing diabetes even before it starts. The most dramatic example comes from a small study in which the onset of type 1 diabetes was delayed several years in high-risk children. In it, brothers and sisters of kids with diabetes injected themselves with a low dose of insulin each day to improve beta-cell function. All twelve children in the study had normal glucose-tolerance tests at the outset. Over the next few years, those at high risk were identified based on specific tests.

"Our study showed that it is possible to predict who is going to get diabetes among high-risk relatives, and that it is possible to introduce interventions so that we can begin to postpone, delay, or even prevent diabetes altogether," says Richard Keller, M.D., one of the study's authors.

There have been other inroads as well. Researchers have found that a pancreatic enzyme known as "64K" stimulates production of antibodies in the blood of many people who eventually develop diabetes. It is not yet clear whether the antibodies play a direct role in destroying insulin-producing cells or whether they are a secondary effect of an autoimmune attack by other cells. In any case, researchers believe they are a sign of impending diabetes. And because this enzyme is the same as an enzyme present in large quantities in the brain, researchers expect that the finding may lead to a simple test to screen for people who are likely to develop the disease years before symptoms appear.

Diabetes Prevention Trials

In the United States and around the world, researchers now are conducting clinical trials to discover whether type 1 diabetes can be prevented in high-risk patients. In fact, two such trials are currently underway at the National Institutes of Health, one examining whether insulin injections will delay diabetes, the other looking into whether eating capsules of crystallized insulin will delay the disease.

People who are the first- or second-degree relative of someone with type 1 diabetes can help researchers learn more about the disease by participating in these trials. To be eligible to participate:

- You must be a first-degree relative (brother, sister, son, daughter, or parent) of someone with type 1 diabetes and be between the ages of three and forty-five, or a second-degree relative (niece, nephew, cousin, grandchild, aunt, uncle, or half-sibling) and be between the ages of three and twenty.

- You must have blood test results that show you to be at high risk for developing diabetes.

- You must be willing to be randomly assigned to one of three groups: the group that takes insulin injections, the group that takes capsules of insulin, or a control group that receives no experimental treatment.

continues

For more information on how to become part of the clinical trials, contact the national coordinating center in Miami at 800-HALT-DM-1.

CURING DIABETES

For those who already have diabetes, doctors are looking into ways to replace beta cells in the pancreas, primarily through transplantation—a surgery that helps treat diabetes.

Today, pancreas transplantation is the only way for people with type 1 diabetes to go off insulin. When the pancreas is replaced, the body once again has enough functioning beta cells to produce insulin. The success of pancreas transplants, however, is fairly limited but getting better. In 1997, University of Minnesota transplantation experts David Sutherland, M.D., and Rainer Gruessner, M.D., reported independence from insulin for more than 80 percent of those having simultaneous pancreas and kidney transplants, for more than 70 percent of those having pancreas transplants, after kidney transplants, and for more than 60 percent of those having only pancreas transplants.

However, not everyone can receive a new pancreas. Doctors are very selective about pancreas transplants. Organ rejection remains a major problem. If the organ received does not closely match a person's own tissues, the immune system will attack it. **Immunosuppressive drugs** help protect the new organ and weaken the rejection response, but they can have debilitating side effects—high blood pressure, fever, low white-blood-cell counts, ulcers, and kidney damage.

Because of the risks of immunosuppressive drugs, many surgeons transplant pancreases only in patients with type 1 diabetes whose kidneys have begun to fail. The pancreas is usually transplanted along with a kidney; pancreas-only transplants are less common.

Anyone interested in pancreatic transplantation should thoroughly discuss the pros and cons with his health care practitioner. A hefty price tag comes with the operation—anywhere from $40,000 to more than $100,000. Beyond that are what doctors call "maintenance" costs of about $10,000 a year. As always, it's best to find a hospital and a surgeon who have plenty of experience with this precise type of surgery. One such place is the Mayo Clinic in Rochester, Minnesota; another is the Joslin Diabetes Center in Falmouth, Massachusetts.

The medical profession is still debating whether a successful pancreas transplant will stop the development of diabetic complications. Some doctors are enthusiastic. A report from Sweden indicates that kidney disease does not come back in patients who receive both a kidney and pancreas transplant, and German researchers report that progression of diabetic eye disease slows and circulation in the small blood vessels of the legs and feet improves after pancreas transplantation.

Other doctors point out that some complications may already have set in by the time a transplant is indicated and that the complications will continue despite the new pancreas.

People interested in transplantation should go to a local hospital library and do some research in the medical journals, then talk to their doctors. In addition, the American Diabetes Association can update consumers on transplantation and where it is being done (see the resources listed at the back of this book).

If a person isn't eligible for a pancreas transplant or doesn't want one, there are two other surgical treatments currently under investigation:

- *Transplantation of parts of the pancreas—the islets, which contain the beta cells that manufacture insulin.* Transplanting the islets makes a person insulin independent for at least several years, according to an article in the *Journal of the American Medical Association.* However, cell rejection is still a problem, and so this surgery is still only experimental. Those people who have islet-cell transplants are part of research studies.

- *Restoration of beta cells.* Researchers at the University of Wisconsin have been transplanting beta cells, obtained from the pancreas of an adult or a fetus, in people undergoing kidney transplants. Again, cell rejection is a problem with this approach, as is true of any organ replacement. However, it is a less invasive method of transplantation.

- *Implantation of bioartificial cells.* Insulin-producing islet cells taken from the pancreas of a rat have shown promise as a treatment for diabetes, according to a Duke University researcher. The cells, which would be transplanted just as beta cells are, are treated to prevent an autoimmune response and cell rejection. The cells have yet to be clinically evaluated.

There is also the possibility of an artificial pancreas. You may have heard about the device invented by a physician at Tufts University School of Medicine. He calls his artificial pancreas an ultrafiltering hybrid organ, and he claims the device shields the beta cells of the pancreas from attack by white blood cells. This device has not been tested, so results of its use—positive or negative—are many years down the road. As things stand now, most people with diabetes do not expect a transplant. They learn to live with the condition.

Until a cure or means of prevention is found, people with type 1 diabetes need to maintain a careful balance of insulin and diet. In the best interests of their health, they need to keep an eye on new treatment methods and be aware of the complications that type 1 diabetes often causes. But the most important step is to work to maintain normal blood-sugar levels. There are lots of ways to do this, as the rest of this book demonstrates.

CHAPTER THREE

Handling Type 2 Diabetes

TYPE 1 DIABETES ARISES SWIFTLY AND CAN BE LIFE THREATENING. AS we said in Chapter 1, type 1 diabetes is caused when the pancreas does not produce insulin. Since the body needs insulin to turn food into energy, people with type 1 diabetes absolutely must take insulin in order to live. Without insulin, people with type 1 are also at risk of ketoacidosis, a deadly buildup of poisons in the bloodstream that can develop in a matter of days. For these reasons, type 1 diabetes is considered to be more severe than type 2.

Yet those with type 2 still have to worry. Despite what the perception may be, type 1 and type 2 diabetes are equally hazardous. Type 2 simply poses a different sort of danger, and that is to long-term health.

By now, you know that people with type 2 diabetes still have the ability to produce insulin, but that insulin no longer functions properly. Type 2 diabetes accounts for about 90 to 95 percent of all cases of diabetes. In the United States, 14.9 million adults have type 2 diabetes—and an estimated one-third of them have the disease but don't know it yet. Working with all these people has given the medical profession plenty of time to find out about the long-term characteristics of this disease.

And it has found that type 2 is more insidious than type 1; meaning that it can proceed undetected for many years. Scientists estimate that the onset of type 2 diabetes can be as quick as four to seven years—or as slow as nine to twelve years. Because the symptoms aren't dramatic, no one notices its presence. Unfortunately, in that time the high sugar levels associated with the diabetes may have set the stage for some serious problems, particularly heart disease and circulatory problems. Someone with diabetes, for example, is twice as likely to have a history of heart attack or stroke than his nondiabetic peers. In fact, the longer someone has the disease, the greater his risk of experiencing a related illness.

It is estimated that 25 percent of the cost of treating diabetes in this country is money spent on treating related conditions and complications—primarily cardiovascular conditions that manifest themselves in heart attacks, hardening of the arteries, and strokes. Circulatory problems, such as poor circulation in the feet, that lead to amputation are also common in type 2 diabetes. New research even suggests that people with type 2 diabetes have a greater risk of developing Alzheimer's disease and colorectal cancer than people without the disease.

Many of the complications of diabetes—strokes, heart attacks, hardening of the arteries, and amputations—are the same ones associated with advanced age. All this is evidence of what we've noted before: Diabetes hastens the wear and tear on many crucial bodily functions. To greatly varying degrees, all people with type 2 diabetes experience this wear and tear.

The degenerative process can be slowed, however, through scrupulous attention to a healthy lifestyle and a strong commitment to maintaining target blood-sugar levels. There are a lucky few who have their blood sugar in such control that it's almost as though they no longer have the disease.

Sad to say, however, there are no guarantees. Someone may be the model of self-care and discipline yet still experience a major complication; another person who has always had zigzagging sugar levels may live to a ripe old age. There's no way around it: Life isn't just. But all the experts are adamant: The time a person with diabetes spends on self-care does indeed help to minimize complications down the road.

What Is Type 2 Diabetes?

In order to really get the message about taking type 2 diabetes seriously, you should know a little more about the mechanics of

Overcoming Undertreatment

Strangely enough, a few members of the medical profession just don't see type 2 diabetes as being as serious as type 1, let alone convey the message to their patients that type 2 diabetes is dangerous. Call it a professional prejudice or old-fashioned ignorance, but it's an attitude that does many patients a great disservice. Perhaps it's a holdover from the early days of the century, before insulin was discovered in 1921, when people with type 1 diabetes died young.

Today, doctors know that type 2 diabetes seems mild and nonthreatening in the short term, but all the while, a slow and steady destruction may be taking place. Nonetheless, vestiges of the early preference for treating type 1 patients still linger in the collective memory of the American medical establishment. In some cases, it manifests itself in the undertreatment of diabetes.

By undertreatment, we mean that both physician and patient don't give diabetes the attention it deserves. Sometimes the complications of type 2 diabetes—high blood pressure or foot infections, for example—get more attention than the disease itself. Naturally, some attention is better than none, but only just a little better. Undertreatment is not likely to halt the slow deterioration that years of elevated blood sugar cause.

All of this information plays up the importance of self-care, of taking responsibility for managing your disease. And as we've hinted, this often means changing your lifestyle. That's what this book is all about—taking charge! Granted, that's not always easy to do. But when you look at the other option—unchecked diabetes and its ultimate consequences—the decision becomes easier to make.

the disease itself. The more the medical world studies type 2 diabetes, the more scientists learn that it works in various ways. Scientists now think type 2 diabetes has several components.

Writing in the journal *Postgraduate Medicine,* Priscilla Hollander, M.D., describes these components as:

- An inability of the pancreas to produce insulin.

- An abnormal production of glucose by the liver.

- Insulin resistance, or a problem with the way insulin functions in the body.

Not everyone who has type 2 diabetes will have all of these components. An individual may have one, two, or three, but the most common component by far is insulin resistance. Virtually all people with type 2 have this form of metabolic malfunction.

Insulin resistance is a term used to describe this situation: The pancreas makes insulin, but for some reason the insulin is not very effective at transferring glucose from the blood into the cells of the body. Sound confusing? Imagine your cells as little orbs powered by that form of sugar known as glucose. On the surface of these orbs are tiny structures, called receptors, that serve as gateways to the cell. In order for a cell to absorb glucose, its gateways must be open. Insulin is the hormone that opens those gates by latching onto the cell at its **receptor sites.**

In people with type 2 diabetes, the number of receptors on each cell may be lower than normal. Second, some of the insulin might not be able to latch onto the receptor sites—in effect, these people's cells are resistant to their body's insulin. Third, the pancreas's insulin-producing capacity declines.

There are other theories to explain the mechanics of type 2 diabetes. However, in the end, the cells don't absorb enough glucose from the bloodstream, so high blood-sugar levels develop.

People with type 2 diabetes have plenty of insulin in their bodies. At times, a person with type 2 diabetes may have above-normal levels of insulin. It may seem strange, but there is an explanation. Think of those beta cells in the pancreas, trained to respond whenever blood sugar goes above a certain level. When blood-sugar levels build up because insulin isn't doing its job well, the beta cells cheerfully pump out more insulin. But still that insulin doesn't get used efficiently.

In some people, a high level of insulin eventually builds up in the blood, a situation that doctors call **hyperinsulinemia.**

Whether hyperinsulinemia is something to worry about is unknown. It's been suggested that insulin itself may contribute over the long term to **vascular** disease—in other words, problems with blood vessels, such as hardening of the arteries, a condition known as **atherosclerosis.** But many doctors point out that such concerns are "based on speculation with little supporting data," in the words of diabetes expert Hollander.

The Causes of Type 2 Diabetes

Now that you know that type 2 diabetes can be caused by several problems related to insulin and blood sugar, you need to understand why people develop these problems in the first place. Scientists have linked type 2 diabetes to two predisposing factors. The first—heredity—is fairly obvious.

Type 2 diabetes often runs in families, suggesting that some genetic trait puts people at greater risk of developing type 2 diabetes. Doctors have theories as to which trait that may be. Scientists at the University of California in San Francisco hypothesize that a newly discovered gene that overproduces protein that makes cells resistant to insulin may underlie the development of diabetes. Other researchers postulate that a defect in the way in which skeletal muscles convert glucose into **glycogen** (the form in which glucose is stored for later use) may be the culprit. Scientists are hoping to locate a diabetes gene so they can turn it off or treat it.

But we need to focus on one key point: You are not born with insulin resistance or type 2 diabetes—but you may be born with the ability to develop type 2 diabetes. And this leads us straight to the next influencing factor: obesity.

Obesity means weighing 20 percent more than your healthy body weight. Intimately related to this is overeating, which in and of itself can exacerbate type 2 diabetes. The more a person eats, the greater insulin production needs to be; insulin production is stimulated each time food is eaten.

Obesity is considered to be the primary trigger for insulin resistance and type 2 diabetes. Approximately 85 percent of people with type 2 diabetes are obese and, in almost all cases, the obesity preceded the development of overt diabetes.

Not all obese people will eventually develop diabetes, although many of them become insulin resistant even though they don't develop the skyrocketing sugar levels of diabetes.

But look at it this way: Being overweight places heavy demands on the body for more insulin and contributes to insulin resistance. A person who, say, needs about 50 units of insulin a day at a normal weight might require as much as 120 units daily to maintain normal blood sugar when overweight. The extra insulin is needed to make up for insulin resistance.

Again, some researchers argue that insulin resistance is an acquired condition, not a condition that people are born with. June Biermann and Barbara Toohey, writing in *The Diabetic's*

Book, carry the point further, arguing that obesity is the disease and diabetes the complication.

Whether or not you agree with that view, researchers have found that both insulin resistance and type 2 diabetes can be largely reversed by successful weight loss. With that in mind, let's move on to treatments.

Treating Type 2 Diabetes

A number of different tactics can keep type 2 diabetes in check. These include lifestyle changes, oral medications, insulin injections, and a combination of methods. Treatments may change and vary with time. Since we just mentioned the benefits of successful weight loss, let's begin our discussion of treatment with the subject of diet.

DIET THERAPY

Diet has been called the cornerstone of treatment for type 2 diabetes. It's generally the first treatment a diabetic person tries. "Diet" is a bit of a tricky word. On the one hand, it means careful attention to the foods you eat. On the other hand, the word conjures up images of short-term, intensive periods of calorie deprivation that may or may not be nutritionally sound.

What most diabetes experts mean by diet is a carefully crafted eating plan—a plan that someone with diabetes can comfortably continue for life. Developed perhaps with the assistance of a dietitian or nutritionist, this eating plan will address not only how much food can be eaten but also the type of food eaten. Following an eating plan to improve blood sugar is known as **diet therapy.**

Diet therapy includes two strategies: calorie control and weight loss. For most people with diabetes, accomplishing both requires a complete change in eating habits—a new way of thinking about food, in effect. We discuss the ins and outs of nutrition for people with diabetes in Chapter 5.

A new eating plan can make quite a difference. For someone with type 2 diabetes who is not overweight, simply controlling calories may be all that's needed to improve blood-sugar levels markedly. For someone who is overweight, the weight loss achieved with a low-calorie diet can produce a major improvement in blood-sugar levels.

If you think about it for a minute, you can see how that works: The moment someone stops overeating, the need for insulin decreases and insulin production slows. (Remember: Insulin production is stimulated each time food is eaten.) Cutting back on food intake can immediately reduce blood-glucose levels. At the same time, the symptoms of diabetes—intense hunger and thirst, fatigue, and frequent urination—begin to disappear within a few days, and even before the person has lost an ounce of weight! It's theorized that these changes happen so quickly because a proper diet helps insulin receptors work more effectively. In a sense, they're not constantly being overwhelmed by calories.

Usually, a specific goal is set for which a person with diabetes should aim. Many years ago, doctors set very modest treatment goals for people with diabetes. At that time, the major thrust was to treat the symptoms of diabetes—particularly polyuria (frequent urination) and excessive thirst—and to lower fasting-blood-sugar levels to under 200 mg/dl. Since then, doctors have learned more about the long-term complications of type 2 diabetes, and so today they encourage their patients to strive for a more ambitious achievement—the same target blood-sugar levels aimed for by people with type 1 diabetes.

Targets vary from person to person. Each person with diabetes and his physician must set a realistic goal. Some doctors set a narrower or slightly different range than we're showing here, according to their philosophy of practice. But as a rule of thumb, targets include blood glucose in the range of 80 to 120 mg/dl in the morning before eating; under 180 mg/dl one to two hours after a meal; and 100 to 140 mg/dl at bedtime. Obviously, these are much lower than the blood-glucose level of 200 mg/dl that was the target years ago. Again, targets should vary, and each diabetic person and his physician must set a realistic goal.

The amount of weight a person needs to lose to see blood-sugar improvements is not as much as you might think. A 10 percent weight loss is the figure we've most often come across. As one physician puts it, the goal of weight loss is to decrease insulin resistance, and a person with diabetes doesn't always have to reach his ideal weight to improve blood-sugar levels.

The point is, any amount of weight loss is good because it immediately decreases the amount of insulin you need.

Many people with type 2 diabetes also have **hypertension** (high blood pressure) and **hyperlipidemia** (a high level of fat in the blood). Both hypertension and hyperlipidemia are associated with an increased risk of heart disease—just what you don't need. In addition, high blood pressure strains the heart, wears down the arteries, and increases the risk of stroke, heart attack, and kidney problems. Hypertension and hyperlipidemia are both affected by the type of foods people eat. In Chapter 5, we discuss the foods that should be avoided to keep blood pressure and blood fats down.

Unfortunately, not enough people are able to control diabetes strictly with diet. Statistics published in *Postgraduate Medicine* paint a rather sobering picture: At the end of one year, only 10 to 20 percent of people with type 2 diabetes are able to bring their blood-glucose levels down to normal through diet. Within five years of diagnosis of their disease, around 90 percent with type 2 diabetes need another treatment method.

EXERCISE THERAPY

No one is quite sure why the success rate with diet is so low. Doctors often say it's primarily because their patients are unable to lose weight or to control the amount of calories ingested. It could be that the success rate would be much higher if more people with diabetes made overall lifestyle changes—for example, if they combined a change in eating habits with an earnest commitment to exercise. Medical textbooks often list exercise as being the second step in the treatment of type 2 diabetes, but ideally it should be part and parcel of diet therapy.

Exercise is important because it helps reduce blood-glucose levels and makes insulin more effective. Exercise also helps people lose weight faster and maintain their lower weight. Further, exercise seems to improve insulin's sensitivity (its ability to work), reduces the dosage requirement or the need for blood-glucose medications, and reduces the risk of cardiovascular disease.

Exercise is recommended for everyone—with or without diabetes. We talk at greater length about it in Chapter 5.

Except in rare cases, people can't control diabetes simply by getting lots of exercise—diet must play a part, as well. Some folks think that as long as they are exercising vigorously and regularly, they can eat as much of anything they want. Wrong! Exercise won't control blood glucose, although it does influence it. As we said before, a sound meal plan forms the cornerstone of all treatment for type 2 diabetes. Everything else must build on that sound base.

ORAL THERAPY

If meal planning, better eating habits, weight loss, and regular exercise do not keep blood sugar in a target range, then most mainstream practitioners recommend using medication (in addition to self-care measures) to lower blood glucose. Referred to as oral hypoglycemic agents, oral hypoglycemics, or oral agents, these pills are also prescribed for those people who for whatever reason are unable or unwilling to control their weight and food intake. The use of these pills is called **oral therapy.**

Oral hypoglycemics are drugs that lower blood-sugar levels. They may do it by increasing the amount of insulin the pancreas secretes, by helping the body use insulin more effectively, or by slowing the release of glucose into the bloodstream; the specific mechanism is different in each family of drugs. People with type 1 diabetes cannot use oral hypoglycemics. These agents work only if the body's beta cells are already producing some insulin. Because the beta cells in people with type 1 diabetes have been irrevocably destroyed, these drugs can do nothing for them. The drugs are also ineffective for people with type 2 diabetes who cannot produce insulin. Testing can determine whether a person's pancreas is producing insulin or not.

Types of Drugs

There are a number of oral hypoglycemic agents available. In the United States, oral agents once came from one chemical family, the sulfonylureas. The first-generation sulfonylureas became available in the 1950s; the second-generation drugs were introduced in 1984. In 1995 and 1996, two other chemical families—the biguanides and the alpha-glucosidase inhibitors—joined the oral-agent arsenal. The year 1997 brought still more options, including thiazolidinediones and meglitinides.

First, let's look at the sulfonylureas, which lower blood-glucose levels by stimulating the pancreas to produce more insulin. Seven sulfonylureas are now on the market. We list them by their generic names and give the usual daily doses for each.

Acetohexamide (Dymelor): 250–1,500 mg

Chlorpropamide (Diabinese, Chlorpropamide): 100–750 mg

Glimepiride (Amaryl): 1–8 mg

Glipizide (Glucotrol, Glipizide): 2.5–4.0 mg

Glyburide (DiaBeta, Glynase, Micronase, Glyburide): 1.25–20 mg

Tolazamide (Tolazamide): 100–1,000 mg

Tolbutamide (Tolbutamide): 500–2,000 mg

Each family of diabetes drugs offers different potential side effects. Anyone who uses a sulfonylurea, for example, is at risk for developing low blood-glucose levels, also known as hypoglycemia. Symptoms include hunger, sweating, shaking, dizziness, confusion, irritability, even nausea.

When using sulfonylureas, it's important to monitor blood sugar several times a day. The thing to watch for is a blood-glucose level of 70 mg/dl or below. At that point, the patient needs to take steps immediately to raise blood-sugar levels. Eating certain foods or injecting glucose are two ways to do this. See Chapter 4 for complete details.

Besides the possibility of low blood sugar, there are other problems with sulfonylureas. In general, sulfonylureas tend to promote weight gain (most people gain four to five pounds), which contributes to the severity of diabetes. A less common occurrence is allergic reaction, indicated by a rash, hives, nausea, vomiting, or cramping. Chlorpropamide, a first-generation sulfonylurea, may react with alcohol to create an excruciating headache, a flushed face, and nausea. There has also been some controversy surrounding studies that indicate certain sulfonylureas may increase the risk of death from cardiovascular disease.

Another oral agent is called **metformin,** from the biguanides chemical family. Metformin causes the liver to release stored glucose more slowly. It appears to lower insulin resistance and lower blood glucose without increasing insulin production. Usual doses are 500 to 2,500 mg.

The initial short-term side effects of metformin include nausea, stomach upset, diarrhea, loss of appetite, and, occasionally, low levels of vitamin B_{12}. These effects occur about 30 percent more often in people taking metformin than in those taking a placebo. Metformin's most serious side effect is **lactic**

acidosis, a rare life-threatening buildup of acid in the blood that may develop in people with heart, kidney, or liver disease. If you have one of those three conditions, you should not take metformin.

A newcomer is **acarbose,** the first member of a new family of drugs called alpha-glucosidase inhibitors. Acarbose slows digestion of food, thus slowing the entry of glucose into the bloodstream and preventing surges in blood-glucose levels right after meal. Usual doses are 50 to 100 mg.

Acarbose appears to have relatively mild side effects, specifically gas (occurring about 45 percent more often than with a placebo), abdominal pain (about 12 percent more often), and diarrhea (about 21 percent more often). Many times these problems are only temporary, occurring when a person first uses the drug. However, doctors generally recommend that people with gastrointestinal ailments not take acarbose.

The good news is that metformin and acarbose don't promote weight gain. Blood-sugar levels may stay more even, too: Research shows that acarbose does not produce hypoglycemia, and metformin causes it only occasionally.

In 1997, the first drug from the meglitinide class came on the market. Called **repaglinide,** the drug is similar to sulfonylureas in that it stimulates the production of insulin by the pancreas. Unlike other drugs, which are taken once a day, repaglinide is taken just before a meal to prevent hypoglycemia. It can be used alone or in conjunction with glucophage if either drug is ineffective on its own. Its notable side effects include weight gain and hypoglycemia. The usual dose is 0.5 to 4 mg daily.

FDA also approved **troglitazone,** a member of the drug family thiazolidinedione, in early 1997. The drug, an insulin sensitizer, works by reducing the body's resistance to insulin and can be used alone or in combination with other drugs. Initial research suggested that the drug could reduce fasting blood-glucose levels by 30 percent without causing hypoglycemia. In many cases, the drug reduces or eliminates the need for insulin in those taking it, experts say. Initial recommended dosage is 400 mg or 600 mg daily if the drug is used alone, and 200 mg if used in a combination with another medication. Troglitazone is usually well tolerated, though it sometimes may cause headaches and weight gain. Practitioners have been advised to use caution if prescribing it for people with heart or liver conditions.

When it was approved, experts heralded troglitazone as a development that would revolutionize the treatment of diabetes. Whether the drug is a breakthrough, however, remains to be seen. Only months after its approval, its manufacturer, Warner-Lambert, issued warnings to practitioners, advising them to watch carefully for liver problems in those on the drug. In December 1997, troglitazone was pulled from the market in England because of serious effects on the liver reported by patients in both the United States and Japan.

FDA, however, says that it "continues to find the benefits outweigh the risks" for those treated appropriately with the drug, and the manufacturer reports that the incidence of liver problems is still well under the 2 percent rate found in studies. Currently, troglitazone is still available in the United States. FDA recommends that patients taking troglitazone have liver-function tests monthly during the first eight months of treatment, bimonthly during the next four months of treatment, and periodically after that.

Also under investigation are drugs that suppress or control appetite and, therefore, enable obese people with type 2 diabetes to improve glycemic control by losing weight. One example is **bromocriptine,** a drug currently approved for the treatment of Parkinson's disease. The drug works by increasing insulin sensitivity and also increasing levels of the brain chemical dopamine, suppressing appetite. In studies, bromocriptine reduced blood-glucose levels by up to 29 mg/dl in patients on a weight-maintenance diet and reduced levels of triglycerides (cholesterol-like substances that contribute to heart disease, a worry for those with diabetes) by up to 43 mg/dl, compared with patients on a diet only. With bromocriptine, 13 percent of the subjects in the studies dropped out because of side effects including nausea, fatigue, headache, and rhinitis. The drug has not yet been submitted for review by FDA for use by people with diabetes.

Special Considerations with Oral Therapy

There are a number of considerations for people who are thinking about oral therapy. Those who decide to use an oral hypoglycemic will need to work out with their physicians how frequently to take it. Some oral agents must be taken more than once a day; others can be taken only once daily. The doctor will set up a schedule.

Oral hypoglycemics work better for some people than others. They work best for people who develop diabetes after age forty, whose disease is newly discovered, and who take fewer than 40 units of insulin a day. In prescribing oral hypoglycemics, doctors take into account the consumer's age, weight, and overall health. Oral agents aren't recommended for pregnant women because the effect on the fetus is not known.

And remember: Just because people take oral glycemics doesn't mean that they do not have to be careful about what they eat. They still have to control calorie intake and eat the right foods! Diet can make or break the success of oral therapy. These drugs won't work if the eating plan is neglected.

Other concerns may arise with oral therapy. In some cases, oral agents react with alcohol, as well as with other drugs. Any drug or medication has the potential to interact with another substance. Cortisone, in particular, has been known to raise blood-sugar levels and make oral hypoglycemic agents less effective. When in doubt, even about nonprescription medicines, people should consult with their health care practitioners or pharmacists.

And again, those using oral therapy may need to adjust their regimens when they're sick. Oral hypoglycemics may lose their effectiveness in people who have an illness. That's because periods of physical stress often create a dramatic jump in blood glucose. By physical stress, we mean those times when a person has a fever, cold, or flu; when someone has a sinus infection or a urinary tract infection; when a person has been injured; or when someone is undergoing surgery. During these times, people with type 2 diabetes are often prescribed insulin (usually human insulin) instead of oral agents. After the illness has passed, they may go back to oral therapy, monitoring blood sugar frequently at the start.

Oral therapy might also fail by simply stopping working. It happens frequently with sulfonylureas. As handy as this therapy is for type 2 diabetes, about half of the people who use sulfonylureas eventually stop within five or six years, simply because the drugs no longer work.

Doctors talk about this problem in terms of **primary** and **secondary failure.** Primary failure happens when the drugs don't work in the first place. This happens about 20 to 30 percent of the time—a fairly substantial number. Secondary failure happens when the drug quits working after it had been used successfully for a while. The failure may be due to an infection, surgery, or severe injury, in which case the patient may once again have success with the drug after the ailment or injury is cleared up. In other cases, blood-glucose levels become elevated out of the blue. No one is quite sure what causes secondary failure, although doctors say it can happen when someone stops exercising or neglects the eating plan.

Secondary failure is a significant problem. Each year, there's a 5 to 10 percent chance that a person on oral therapy will experience secondary failure. The medical world hoped that the second-generation sulfonylureas would be less vulnerable to this problem, but that doesn't seem to be the case, although results are still coming in on these new drugs.

When an oral agent fails, a physician may increase the dose or prescribe another. The patient may have better luck with a second drug. But when all appropriate oral hypoglycemics fail, insulin is the next step for some individuals. Others try a form of treatment called **combination therapy,** which we discuss in a moment.

INSULIN THERAPY

Though many people think of insulin therapy as only for those with type 1 diabetes, insulin is used for those with type 2 when other therapies have failed. And to be quite honest, many therapies for diabetes fail, at least according to the medical profession's point of view.

The Estrogen–Diabetes Connection

Although most cases of diabetes in women occur after menopause, no link has ever been found between the hormone estrogen and the development of the condition. However, researchers have now found that estrogen replacement therapy may be a valuable tool in helping prevent the condition and in lowering blood-sugar levels if it does strike.

A survey of some 400 women in Milwaukee conducted by the University of Wisconsin found that women who did not take estrogen therapy after menopause had five times the risk of developing type 2 diabetes than those who took the drugs. And a review of more than 14,000 women from the Northern California Kaiser Permanente Diabetes Registry found that women taking hormone replacement had lower levels of blood sugar than those who did not take it.

The theories as to why estrogen affects diabetes differ. Some researchers feel the hormones help shift body fat distribution in women from the abdomen to the hips—a plus since abdominal fat is a risk factor for diabetes. Others feel estrogen helps reduce insulin resistance and improves the function of the beta cells in the pancreas.

Estrogen therapy isn't for everyone, but women with diabetes may want to take the research into account when making their decision. "When women with diabetes assess the pros and cons

continues

97

of estrogen replacement therapy based on their own personal risk profile, these findings may be a factor to take into consideration and discuss with their physicians," said Leslie O. Schultz, professor and chair of health sciences at the University of Wisconsin, one of the researchers on the Milwaukee survey.

Diabetes expert Priscilla Hollander, M.D., explains it this way: If achieving normal blood-sugar levels is the treatment goal for type 2, then the United States has a fairly dismal track record. "Only a fraction of patients do well on diet therapy alone," she writes in *Postgraduate Medicine*. "Eventually, 60 to 70 percent of patients with type 2 diabetes who are being treated aggressively need insulin treatment."

Injected insulin helps with type 2 diabetes because it gives beta cells in the pancreas a rest—after all, the disease has been forcing them to work overtime. After a period of time, when blood sugar has been controlled, the patient may be able to resume the use of oral agents.

Unfortunately, there are a few drawbacks to giving insulin to patients with type 2 diabetes. The first is hyperinsulinemia, the buildup of high levels of insulin in the blood. Giving insulin to insulin-resistant type 2 patients may contribute to or worsen hyperinsulinemia, which may be a risk factor for cardiovascular disease.

Another area of concern with insulin therapy is its effectiveness in very overweight people. Some extremely obese people with type 2 diabetes require huge amounts of insulin, and even with large doses, they aren't able to control their blood sugar. In addition, insulin tends to promote weight gain, a particularly undesirable effect for type 2 patients, as most of them are overweight to begin with. However, these problems are not common.

Insulin therapy may be best for those with type 2 diabetes who have poor control over their blood-sugar levels. A 1997 study from the Type II Diabetes Patient Outcomes Research Team found that people with poor control of diabetes improved their blood-sugar levels substantially with the use of insulin; however, for those who already had moderate control of blood sugar, a switch to insulin didn't lower levels that much more.

To find out more about how to use insulin, we recommend that you read Chapter 2 of this book, which reviews the ins and outs of insulin injection. Most people with type 2 diabetes on insulin need to take two shots of it a day, just like their type 1 peers. Many do well taking a mixture of regular (short-acting insulin) and NPH (intermediate-acting insulin) twice a day—oftentimes before breakfast and dinner—which is again similar to the most common regimen used by people with type 1 diabetes.

Anyone with diabetes—type 1 or type 2—using insulin must monitor blood-glucose levels several times a day. The data derived from these blood-glucose readings provide the physician and person with diabetes with the information needed to make adjustments in insulin doses and to watch for instances of hypoglycemia—a common problem with insulin use.

Combination Therapy

Combination therapy, as the name suggests, combines two different medications, such as a sulfonylurea with metformin, acarbose, insulin, or troglitazone. One of the benefits of this mix-and-match approach is that the medication program can be tailored to the patient. Also, smaller doses of medication, particularly insulin, may be more effective in combination than when used alone. Indeed, a Finnish study found that type 2 patients treated with insulin and sulfonylurea required 50 percent less insulin compared with an insulin-only group.

Combination therapy is used when an oral agent on its own fails or when a patient reaches the maximum dose of an oral agent and still can't control blood sugar.

Surgical Procedures for Diabetes

There are two surgical procedures that can affect diabetes, but they are not really treatments for diabetes: gastric stapling and vertical banding gastroplasty. Both procedures do the same thing—they make a small pouch out of part of the stomach, thereby shrinking the size of it.

Theoretically, the person who has such surgery cannot eat as much food as before. Because these procedures affect food intake, they affect diabetes. But, to reiterate, they are not "surgical cures" for diabetes.

Doctors are debating the role of pancreas transplants, beta-cell transplants, and/or use of an artificial pancreas for type 2 diabetes—the same sort of surgical approaches to type 1 diabetes now in clinical investigation and which we talked about in Chapter 2. But those aren't options for type 2 diabetes right now, although they may be in the future. The best tools for handling the disease still remain the most fundamental ones: diet and exercise.

It ultimately all comes back to diet. While some with diabetes will always struggle with high blood-sugar levels, there's no reason more people cannot succeed at maintaining target levels through a combination of weight loss, careful eating, and exercise. Remember: One-fifth of everyone with type 2 diabetes has succeeded at controlling blood sugar through diet. This doesn't mean their diabetes is gone forever, but as long as they maintain a healthy weight and stick with their eating plan, their blood-glucose levels stay normal, although their blood-sugar levels may creep up every once in a while.

For many folks, shedding pounds enables them to wave goodbye to diabetes and its many related conditions, such as high blood pressure and cardiovascular disease. Diabetic complications are the subject of our next chapter.

CHAPTER FOUR

Diabetic Complications

MOST PEOPLE WITH DIABETES EXPERIENCE COMPLICATIONS. DIABETES has widespread impact, reaching into every corner of the body and touching every system. Its effects are cumulative; particularly vulnerable are the eyes, the heart, the blood vessels, and the feet.

There was a time in the not too distant past when diabetes was devastating. Many people with diabetes died young; others were crippled by one or another of the disease's major complications, such as blindness and kidney failure, and by amputation. Then insulin was discovered in 1921, and people with diabetes had a tool to help keep the more debilitating complications in check. Today we know that through careful lifestyle choices, people can delay the onset of diabetic complications and slow the progression of the disease and its related ailments.

Despite these inroads, diabetic complications remain a reality for some folks. And in that lies a certain irony: Medical science now helps people with diabetes live longer, but the longer they have the disease, the greater their risk of experiencing any of a variety of conditions related to the disease.

Eye disease is one such condition. Diabetes is the major cause of blindness in adults: Blindness is five times more prevalent among people with diabetes than among people with normal blood-sugar levels. Infections and ulcers in the lower legs and feet are other diabetes-related problems. Diabetes is responsible for half of the amputations performed in the United States. In addition, diabetes is thought to cause a quarter of kidney failures. And people with diabetes experience heart attacks and strokes twice as often as people who don't have diabetes.

How these complications develop is the subject of this chapter.

The Factors Behind Complications

Generally, you can't tell diabetic complications are developing, at least not without undergoing tests or medical procedures in a doctor's office. Diabetes proceeds unnoticed, silently ravaging the body. You might be without symptoms until some damage is already done.

There is, however, one surefire indication that problems are developing: persistently high blood-sugar levels. Diabetes experts believe that over the long haul levels above 240 mg/dl are unacceptable and dangerous. However, the ideal level for you is the target set by you and your physician. It will probably be in the 80 to 120 mg/dl range.

The length of time a person has diabetes also comes into play when looking at complications. Because people with type 1 diabetes usually get the disease earlier in life than those with type 2, they have the dubious distinction of running a greater risk of developing complications than those with type 2. For the most part, complications appear in people who have had diabetes for fifteen years or more, although certain short-term complications can appear (and disappear) at any time. Evidence of diabetes-related eye problems, for example, is present after five years in 1 percent of type 1 cases; by fourteen years, the percentage is close to 100.

The type of complications that develop also depends on diabetes type. Individuals with type 1 tend to develop different problems than those with type 2. For instance, type 1 diabetes tends to produce vision problems sooner than does type 2 diabetes, while type 2 diabetes appears to be linked to more heart attacks and strokes. The rates at which complications proceed also vary wildly.

Scientists don't really know why these differences exist. Nor do they know why complications sometimes develop in people who have blood-sugar levels firmly in hand while other people never develop complications, regardless of how well or how poorly they control their blood sugar. It may boil down to genetic differences or even to factors yet unknown.

There are somewhere in the neighborhood of three dozen kinds of diabetic complications out there, if you count various small conditions and infections. It may be more helpful, however, to look at these problems as falling into two groups.

Diabetic complications are classified as short term (those that strike quickly at any time) and long term (those that develop only after someone has had diabetes for years). The medical profession often uses the term **acute** when talking of short-term, rapidly occurring complications and **chronic** when referring to long-term complications. Let's take a look at these two types of complications now.

Short-Term Complications

Short-term complications are no less serious than long-term problems. They can occur at any time and can certainly be dangerous, sometimes fatal. But the plus side of short-term problems (if you can think of problems as being positive!) is that they generally can be prevented or reversed. The most common are hypoglycemia and diabetic ketoacidosis, or coma.

HYPOGLYCEMIA

Hypoglycemia, as we've mentioned before, is a dangerously low level of blood sugar. Usually indicated by blood-glucose readings of 70 mg/dl or lower, hypoglycemia is one of the most common complications of diabetes, which people often call an insulin reaction.

How It Happens

Hypoglycemia begins abruptly, and once the cycle of low blood sugar gets under way, it can proceed rapidly. In a matter of hours, a person may go from feeling uncomfortable to becoming irritable and incoherent. The latter are signals that the brain is no longer getting enough glucose. Eventually, if the low sugar levels continue, the person may pass out and go into a coma. Left untreated, hypoglycemia can cause death.

Doctors sometimes call hypoglycemia an **iatrogenic** condition, meaning that it can be caused by the *treatment* of the disease. To understand how treatment can cause this condition, consider the situation of someone with untreated diabetes: Her blood sugar is always above normal, so she isn't at risk of hypoglycemia, or low blood sugar. Once someone begins to treat her diabetes—in other words, use diet, exercise, insulin, or medications (oral agents) to maintain blood sugar at normal or near-normal levels—then she is more likely to have instances when she overshoots the mark, so to speak, and brings her blood sugar down too far.

Insulin reactions frequently happen to people who use insulin or oral hypoglycemic agents, and they're especially prevalent in those people with type 1 diabetes who follow a regimen of tight blood-glucose control. (See the discussion of tight control in Chapter 2 for more details.) As you recall, achieving a normal blood-sugar level is a delicate balance between sugar and insulin. Too much insulin can upset the applecart.

To be very specific, someone might take too much insulin or too large a dose of an oral hypoglycemic agent. If the overdose is not counterbalanced, very low blood-sugar levels may develop.

There are, of course, other ways that someone taking insulin or oral agents might inadvertently cause blood-sugar levels to fall too far. They include delaying or skipping a meal, not eating enough carbohydrates in a meal, and exercising too much, unexpectedly, or at the wrong time of day. Drinking a large quantity of alcohol can sometimes throw blood-sugar levels out of whack.

Recognizing the Signs

Early symptoms of hypoglycemia include weakness, trembling, intense hunger, cold and clammy skin, sweating, quick pulse, headache, anxiety, and irritability. Later symptoms include headache, confusion, and drowsiness. In severe cases, unconsciousness or seizures may occur. (Of course, not everyone will experience all of these symptoms; in fact, some may not experience symptoms at all, which we discuss in a minute.) Treating severe insulin reactions requires assistance from another person, as the affected person can no longer help herself.

These may sound like fairly clear-cut symptoms, and for most people they serve sufficient warning. Unfortunately, many people experience a situation called **reaction denial.** This occurs when a person refuses to admit to an insulin reaction; usually, the person can no longer think clearly because blood-glucose levels in the brain are too low—sometimes 20 or 30 mg/dl. In such cases, a friend or family member must cajole the person into drinking something sugary, such as soda, to get sugar levels up. After the insulin reaction is over, the person often looks back and says, "Yes, you were right. I did need more sugar."

There's a similar problem that isn't exactly reaction denial. It's sometimes referred to as **hypoglycemic unawareness.** This happens when people *don't experience* those warning signals. Those people with type 1 diabetes who follow a tight-control regimen are most likely to have this problem. One team of Australian researchers studied such individuals and found that their subjects couldn't detect the warning signs of hypoglycemia 64 percent of the time when using human insulin and 69 percent of the time when using pork-derived insulin.

We've come across two explanations as to why some people don't experience symptoms. The first attributes it to the fact that when someone maintains blood sugar at near-normal levels, a drop from, say, 85 mg/dl to 60 mg/dl is not very dramatic and therefore, less noticeable than, say, a drop from 240 mg/dl to 60 mg/dl that a person with unstable diabetes might experience.

Researchers offer a more technical explanation: the absence of a hormone called **glucagon.** Glucagon is a naturally occurring substance found in the blood, one of several so-called counter-regulatory hormones that help keep the body's sugar and insulin levels on an even keel. (Another of these counter-regulatory hormones is **epinephrine,** otherwise known as adrenaline.) Glucagon is secreted by the pancreas, and its role is to raise blood-sugar levels when those levels get too low.

Recently, scientists have found that most people with type 1 diabetes slowly and gradually lose the ability to produce glucagon in response to low blood-sugar levels. This problem seems to develop during the first five years of the disease. Without this "glucagon response" to low blood sugar, people with diabetes are at high risk of severe hypoglycemic reactions, particularly with a tight-control insulin regimen. These people often no longer experience anxiety, shaking, or other warning signals and don't realize they have hypoglycemia.

Since hypoglycemia can cause reaction denial and hypoglycemic unawareness, there's only one way to find out whether you have it: Take a blood-glucose reading. Using a home blood-glucose measurement kit and following the guidelines for self-monitoring of blood glucose (SMBG), you can get the real lowdown on the state of your sugar levels. Readings from the kit's blood-glucose meter can disclose what your mood or symptoms cannot. (We've mentioned SMBG in previous chapters, and we thoroughly discuss this all-important self-care technique in Chapter 5.)

Handling the Problem

Once you realize hypoglycemia has developed—either with the help of a glucose meter or because of symptoms—steps need to be taken to bring blood-sugar levels back up. Many doctors recommend that you eat or drink something with carbohydrates when sugar levels get to 70 mg/dl. Below 60 mg/dl, you should treat the situation like a medical emergency—because it could well be. Again, the first step to recovery is to eat or drink something. Traditional recommendations include drinking a small glass of fruit juice or a soft drink with sugar or eating dried fruit, six or seven Lifesavers, two tablespoons of raisins, six jelly beans, or several glucose tablets.

Once the reaction is treated, you may need to eat an additional small meal, a snack, or a pharmaceutically developed food product (such as the Zbar food bar) to prevent blood sugar from dropping again later in the day.

Your health care practitioner can give you additional guidelines for treating insulin reactions, including a list of foods to keep close at hand. It's a good idea for anyone prone to hypoglycemia to carry a small amount of sugary foods to be eaten in the event of an insulin reaction. You might also tell people around you what to do should you develop a serious reaction.

If a person doesn't get blood-sugar levels up soon enough, he may become disoriented, confused, or even unconscious. Since you can't give food or drink by mouth to someone who is unconscious (the person may choke to death), someone will have to inject glucagon.

Glucagon, which was mentioned earlier in connection to hypoglycemia, is a naturally occurring hormone that works to regulate blood-sugar levels. Like the hormone insulin, glucagon is manufactured by pharmaceutical companies for use by people with diabetes, and, again like insulin, it is injected with syringe and needle. A glucagon injection is the way to treat a person who is unconscious because of **insulin shock.**

To prevent insulin reactions, you can monitor blood-sugar levels frequently and act accordingly. But it's nigh on to impossible to go through life with diabetes and not experience several insulin reactions.

KETOACIDOSIS

Ketoacidosis, commonly called a diabetic coma, primarily affects people with type 1 diabetes. (People with type 2 diabetes experience another form of diabetic coma, and we discuss that in a moment.) Ketoacidosis is caused by a persistently high level of blood sugar, or hyperglycemia.

Certain situations enable hyperglycemia to grab a foothold: too much food; not enough exercise; not enough insulin or medication; physical stress, such as an infection, the flu, or another illness; and psychological stress.

A coma is a serious proposition. Before insulin was discovered, ketoacidosis was a leading cause of death in people with diabetes. Even today people who do not control their diabetes can die from a diabetic coma. However, most people learn to recognize and treat the early stages of this complication, thus avoiding its tragic repercussions.

How It Happens

Ketoacidosis usually comes on slowly, over the course of many days. The situation develops like this:

- Blood sugar builds up when the cells cannot absorb glucose for use as energy. At this point, the body begins to burn fat as fuel, producing waste products known as **ketones.** These ketones accumulate in the blood (a situation known as **ketosis**) and eventually work their way into the urine (a situation known as **ketonuria**).

- As ketones continue to build up, a tremendous amount of fluid (in the form of urine) is discharged from the body and dehydration begins. The blood eventually becomes extremely acidic. At this point, ketoacidosis has set in. If untreated, ketoacidosis affects brain function, leading to loss of consciousness and death.

- It might take twelve hours, it might take thirty-six, but ketoacidosis is a certainty if the person doesn't recognize his symptoms and take steps to lower his blood glucose.

Recognizing the Signs

The symptoms may include frequent urination and great thirst, vomiting and nausea, blurred vision, abdominal pain, disorientation, and drowsiness. Unconsciousness finally results.

When the person notices symptoms that resemble those of ketoacidosis, the first step is to test his blood-sugar levels. If those levels are over 240 mg/dl, the next step is to test the urine for the presence of ketones. Ketones are sometimes referred to as **acetones,** and the urine test for ketones is sometimes called a urine acetone test.

If both blood-sugar and ketone levels are high, the person should call his physician. In most cases, additional insulin doses can rein in this condition before it reaches the advanced stage— when ketoacidosis must be treated in a hospital.

Handling the Problem

Hospital care is necessary with advanced ketoacidosis because special care is needed to replace body fluids and treat the body for shock. Further, health care practitioners can monitor blood glucose and other blood chemicals much more easily in a hospital setting, giving additional doses of insulin when needed. Minerals such as potassium are often very low and must be replaced gradually. When the person's blood chemistry returns to normal, he can resume his normal self-care regimen.

Coma can occur as ketoacidosis advances, but actually, the moniker *diabetic coma* is misleading: You don't have to be unconscious to have ketoacidosis. Obviously, it's not a good idea to let it get to an advanced stage. Any of the symptoms, plus ketones in the urine, are signals to take immediate action. You can avoid a coma and even hospitalization from this short-term complication by acting quickly when blood-sugar levels are high. You can find out your levels through self-testing.

Hyperosmolar, or Nonketotic, Coma

For people with type 2 diabetes, a different form of coma may be experienced. It's known as the **hyperosmolar, or nonketotic, coma.** We should note here that some people don't distinguish between ketoacidosis and hyperosmolar comas because the symptoms are similar and both are caused by high sugar levels. However, the hyperosmolar coma has a different chemical basis.

How It Happens

In simple terms, in a hyperosmolar coma, ketones do not develop as they do in a diabetic coma—thus the name, nonketotic coma. Insulin is present in the person with type 2 diabetes, and even though it cannot work properly, it prevents the body from burning fat as an alternative fuel. If fat isn't burned, then ketones aren't produced—thus, the chemical difference between ketoacidosis and the hyperosmolar coma.

The cause of both comas—high blood-sugar levels—is the same, however. In a person who is insulin resistant, the body tries to lower blood-glucose levels by filtering the blood through the kidneys, which causes the kidneys to work overtime and also causes frequent urination. A tremendous amount of fluid may be lost, causing dehydration. Although the blood doesn't become acidic, as is the case with ketoacidosis, it becomes concentrated, which is just as dangerous. Blood concentration due to dehydration is described as hyperosmolar, which means "increased concentration of blood."

Recognizing the Signs

The symptoms are similar to those of ketoacidosis: frequent urination and great thirst, nausea, abdominal pain, dry skin, disorientation, and later, labored breathing and drowsiness. And like ketoacidosis, a person need not actually be in a coma to be experiencing a hyperosmolar coma—although that person will probably be disoriented and confused.

Handling the Problem

To treat this condition, it's important to test blood-glucose levels regularly. If they are unusually high for several tests in a row, more insulin or medication may be called for. *The Joslin Diabetes Manual* recommends that you get immediate medical assistance when your blood sugar remains over 400 mg/dl for twelve straight hours despite additional doses of insulin. Once dehydration sets in, you may have to be hospitalized so that liquids, sugars, and other blood chemicals can be stabilized.

You may have noticed that insulin reactions, caused by very low blood sugar, and diabetic comas, caused by very high blood sugar, are difficult to tell apart. However, in the early phases of each there are differences. In general, an insulin reaction tends to appear abruptly. The person is sweaty, with moist, clammy skin, and is nervous and edgy. Diabetic comas develop over a period of days. Someone with an impending coma will have dry skin and nausea and will be drowsy or dazed.

The thing to remember is that everyone has different responses to high and low blood sugar, so you may want to know what their symptoms tend to be. Self-monitoring of blood glucose can track sugar patterns and guard against these short-term, but potentially deadly, complications.

Long-Term Complications

Long-term, chronic complications differ from short-term complications in that they take more time in developing, and once they arrive are less likely to disappear. Many long-term complications are tied to those structures that distribute blood throughout the body: the small and large blood vessels. Although scientists are not certain how it happens, they think that years of carrying blood with high sugar levels eventually damages or impairs blood vessels. The faulty metabolism of someone with diabetes may also create some chemical change that makes blood vessels more vulnerable to damage. Either way, many diabetic complications are vascular complications—complications pertaining to blood vessels, in other words.

Let's look now at some of the major long-term complications faced by people with diabetes.

EYE PROBLEMS

Eye problems that diabetes might cause include minor problems in focusing, premature development of **cataracts,** and various degrees of retinal damage (otherwise known as diabetic retinopathy).

If you have diabetes, it's very likely that you will experience at least one of these problems in the course of your lifetime. Most people who have had diabetes for five to ten years show some signs of eye damage, although it may be slight.

Cataracts

A cataract, a clouding of the lens in the eye, is a very common problem in older people, including folks who don't have diabetes. However, the evidence suggests that diabetes accelerates cataract development. The hastened development is thought to be a result of the intricate and still incompletely understood relationship between high blood-sugar levels and aging. One popular theory posits that when people have diabetes for an extended period of time, sugar by-products begin to build up in the lens of the eye, eventually leading to cataracts.

Mild cataracts are often left as they are—but an individual with diabetes is encouraged to work at keeping blood-sugar levels within the normal range, which seems to slow the accumulation of sugar by-products and, thus, slow the progression of complications.

Once severe cataracts develop, however, many **ophthalmologists** believe that the best course of action is to remove the cataract and replace it with an artificial lens, also known as an **intraocular lens.** This surgical procedure can be done right in a doctor's office.

Although cataracts certainly impede good vision, they are less troublesome than another long-term complication, diabetic retinopathy.

Diabetic Retinopathy

Diabetic retinopathy means damage to or disease of the retina, the delicate membrane that lines the inside wall of the eye. The retina responds to light and receives the image formed by the lens. When it becomes seriously damaged, blindness may result. In fact, retinopathy is the most frequent cause of vision loss in Americans 20 to 74 years old.

Diabetic retinopathy is caused by changes or abnormalities in the small blood vessels of the retina—changes that take years to occur. Experts estimate that 6,000 people a year develop retinopathy. Fortunately, early diagnosis and prompt treatment often can prevent blindness.

Almost everyone with diabetes develops this complication, but the first to feel its impact are people with type 1 diabetes, who frequently develop a mild form of this condition within five years of diagnosis of diabetes. In fact, there's a strong correlation between the amount of time someone has diabetes and the development of retinopathy. Quite simply, the longer you have diabetes, the greater your chance of developing retinopathy. Within ten years of diabetes diagnosis, half of all people with type 1 diabetes and a quarter with type 2 have some damage to their retinas. By twenty years after diagnosis of diabetes, nearly everyone with type 1 diabetes and over 60 percent with type 2 have some degree of retinopathy.

Retinopathy is not something to ignore. Among those with type 1 diabetes, retinopathy is responsible for four-fifths of all cases of blindness; among those with type 2, the number is one-third. Of course, not all cases of retinopathy result in blindness. The condition ranges in severity from mild to advanced.

The medical profession describes two forms of diabetic retinopathy: **background retinopathy** and **proliferative retinopathy.** Background retinopathy is a mild, early form of retinopathy that is characterized by gradual narrowing or weakening of the small blood vessels in the eye. Small bulges (called **microaneurysms**) develop on the vessels. Eventually a vessel may tear or break and then bleed (known in medical parlance as a **hemorrhage**).

Most folks with diabetes develop background retinopathy, but in the lion's share of the cases, the condition remains at a mild level. Vision is not affected unless blood vessels break and leak fluid into the **macula,** an area of the retina responsible for sharp, fine vision—the kind of vision needed to read this book. When fluid leaks into the macula, it swells and puts pressure on other areas of the eye. This situation is called a **macular edema** and it leads to blurred vision. The swelling is sometimes treated in people who appear to be at high risk for blindness with a high-tech procedure known as **photocoagulation.** In this, a precise laser beam is used to sear shut the leaking blood vessels. Photocoagulation doesn't cure retinopathy, but it can delay the loss of vision by a number of years or, in some cases, stop progression.

For the most part, however, because background retinopathy is mild, surgical treatment isn't necessary.

Proliferative retinopathy, as its name suggests, is a severe form of retinopathy that develops when a network of new, fragile blood vessels proliferates in the retina at the site of previous breakages or hemorrhages. The new vessels are an attempt by the eye to repair the damaged, worn-out vessels caused by diabetes. Over time the new, fragile vessels may tear and leak blood into the **vitreous humor,** the clear, gelatinous material that fills the center of the eye. A small amount of blood won't dim vision, but the major hemorrhages associated with proliferative retinopathy may be large enough to affect sight, in which case they are known as **vitreous hemorrhages.**

As the eye tries to repair the damage caused by hemorrhages, scar tissue forms. The buildup of scar tissue may eventually damage the retina, resulting in partial loss of sight, or it may displace or cause the retina to become detached, resulting in total loss of vision.

It may be difficult to tell if either form of retinopathy is developing. For the most part, people can have severe eye damage without knowing it, because the damage may not affect vision and may cause no pain. Of course, there are some obvious indications to the person with diabetes that something has happened to the eye. Partial loss of vision—even if very small—is an indication of a problem. "Floaters," "cobwebs," and "cotton wool balls" are terms that people have used to describe vision problems caused by tiny hemorrhages in the eye. A sudden, painful loss of vision may indicate a major hemorrhage.

Naturally, it's best to detect retinopathy before it reaches this stage. Eye examinations with a tool called a monocular direct ophthalmoscope are used to detect damage to the retina. A family physician can perform this test, although several studies indicate that physicians who are not ophthalmologists detect proliferative retinopathy in only 50 percent of the people who have the condition. That's not a particularly encouraging track record—"No better than random chance," in the words of one eye expert.

There are some treatment options for those people with advanced stages of either form of retinopathy. Photocoagulation—the use of laser beams—can seal leaking retinal blood vessels or reattach a detached retina. In some people, this is enough to stop the progression of diabetic retinopathy.

Vitrectomy is another, more intricate surgical procedure used in people with proliferative retinopathy. In this procedure, a physician removes the vitreous to clear out the light-blocking hemorrhage, uses microsurgery to repair the retina, if necessary, and then replaces the vitreous with a saline solution.

An article in the journal *Annals of Internal Medicine* explains that photocoagulation and vitrectomy prevent deterioration of vision in around 60 percent of patients. Laser therapy reportedly reduces the rate of vision loss by 50 percent in people with proliferative retinopathy and macular edema, conditions that often exhibit no symptoms. Vitrectomy reportedly improves visual acuity to 10/20 or better in 36 percent of treated eyes. That's the good news.

However, no surgery is free of potential complications. With vitrectomy, for example, the overall complication rate is about 25 percent, according to the *Annals of Internal Medicine* article. Potential complications include infection, cataract development, bleeding, elevated pressure in the eye (which can lead to a condition called glaucoma), loss of vision, and retinal detachment or scarring.

Medical research is also looking at ways of slowing or even preventing the progression of retinopathy. One small Norwegian study found that people with type 1 diabetes who maintained near-normal levels of blood sugar over a long period of time—at least seven years—were significantly less likely to develop severe retinopathy. The patients in this study followed a tight-control regimen, using either continuous subcutaneous infusion pumps or multiple insulin injections. (See the discussion of tight control in Chapter 2 for a refresher in what this regimen entails.)

The results of the Diabetes Control and Complications Trial show that tight blood-sugar control can prevent new cases of retinopathy. Tight control also helps retinopathy from growing worse. According to the study, the earlier tight control is instituted, the more beneficial it is at fending off complications.

Scientists are also hoping to discover why high levels of blood glucose damage the body's blood vessels. One theory is that an enzyme called **aldose reductase,** which converts glucose into a sugar alcohol called **sorbitol,** may play a role in triggering diabetic complications. For that reason researchers are looking into a class of drugs called **aldose reductase inhibitors** that block the actions of the enzyme. They hope these drugs can reduce the chance of developing retinopathy and other long-term complications. Studies are underway.

In November 1997, the *Journal of the American Medical Association* reported on a number of other agents that may potentially prevent retinopathy. These include aminoguanidine, a drug that inhibits the formation of certain proteins and lipids that are thought to contribute to blood vessel damage. Other possibilities include drugs that interfere with the growth of blood vessels in the retina; antioxidants such as vitamin E, thought to prevent damage to the endothelium (the innermost layer of the cornea, the clear covering of the eye); and agents that would interfere with the molecular and cellular reactions within the eye that cause cell death.

Although these new treatments sound promising, the key action in the here and now is getting prompt medical care for retinopathy, particularly if you have macular edema or proliferative retinopathy. Studies have found that there is a 16 percent risk for severe visual loss if proliferative retinopathy is left untreated for two years. That may sound like a small risk, but is it really one that's worth taking? You and your doctor must decide.

There are other ways diabetes can exacerbate retinopathy. Poor blood-sugar control, high blood pressure, and a history of smoking increase the risk of retinopathy and increase the chances that the condition will worsen. And as we mentioned before, people with type 1 diabetes are more likely to develop severe retinopathy.

A woman with type 1, type 2, or gestational diabetes who has no retinopathy before pregnancy is unlikely to develop retinopathy during pregnancy. However, the story is different for women with diabetes who already have some retinal damage when they become pregnant. About 5 to 12 percent of women with diabetes with mild retinopathy will see their retinopathy worsen. Women who already have moderate to severe diabetic retinopathy are at greater risk during pregnancy. In recent studies, about 47 percent of pregnant women with diabetes had an increase in severity in retinal damage, and 5 percent developed proliferative retinopathy.

These rapid changes may be due to the increased levels of hormones that accompany pregnancy. Pregnancy-induced or chronic high blood pressure is thought to play a role, too. In one study, 55 percent of pregnant women with diabetes who had high blood pressure in addition to retinopathy saw their retinopathy worsen, compared with 25 percent of the women who had normal blood pressure and retinopathy.

Experts say that pregnant women with signs of retinal damage can slow the progression of retinopathy by lowering blood-pressure levels. Doctors have also found that treating a woman's retinopathy with photocoagulation can help reduce the risk of progression if the laser treatment is done before she becomes pregnant.

Like anyone with diabetic retinopathy, pregnant women should get regular eye examinations to monitor the course and development of this complication.

NEPHROPATHY

Officially known as diabetic nephropathy, nephropathy is a type of kidney disease that leads to kidney failure. Nephropathy tends to develop in people who have had diabetes for 20 years or more. It used to be that a third of all people with type 1 diabetes developed nephropathy, but today's treatment methods and the emphasis on better blood-sugar control are shrinking that percentage. People with type 2 diabetes develop nephropathy infrequently.

How It Happens

To see why nephropathy would be a problem, let's look first at what the kidneys do. The kidneys are organs located near the waist. Inside the kidneys are small blood vessels, called **glomeruli,** that act as filters, removing wastes from the blood and discharging them through the urine. Useful products, such as protein and glucose, are not eliminated but are sent back into the bloodstream.

Nephropathy is the condition in which small arteries in the kidneys become hardened and the glomeruli become damaged, in much the same way that the small vessels of the eye become damaged during retinopathy. The kidneys ultimately fail in their job of filtering out wastes. People with kidney failure must go on **dialysis** (the use of a machine to filter blood) or have a kidney transplant; otherwise, lethal levels of wastes and toxins build up in their bodies.

Nephropathy is caused by high blood-sugar levels. Also, high blood pressure, **arteriosclerosis,** smoking, and high cholesterol increase the likelihood of kidney complications. Frequent urinary tract infections add to the problem because an infection can easily spread to the kidneys and damage them.

Recognizing the Signs

Early warning signs of nephropathy include problems emptying the bladder, blood in the urine, and urinary tract infections. The disease can be confirmed through simple urine and blood tests. Just as the kidneys lose their ability to discharge wastes, they also lose their ability to keep protein and glucose in circulation. Sugar and protein begin to show up in the urine tests in larger and larger amounts. Blood tests also detect high levels of urea nitrogen and creatinine, another indication of kidney damage.

Handling the Problem

To halt kidney damage before kidney failure occurs, the wisest step is to take urinary tract infections seriously. Remember: Infections can back up further into the urinary system and spread to the kidneys, impairing their function.

If signs of developing kidney problems are detected, doctors often recommend a regimen of tight blood-sugar control and a low-protein diet (see Chapter 5) to ease stress on the kidneys. Recent clinical studies suggest that use of the blood-pressure drug enalapril (Vasotec) may preserve kidney function, but more research is needed to confirm this.

CARDIOVASCULAR DISEASE

The word **cardiovascular** means "of the heart and blood vessels." Cardiovascular complications include problems such as angina, heart attack, stroke, and others related to poor circulation. Cardiovascular disease is the most common complication of type 2 diabetes. In fact, people with diabetes have a risk of cardiovascular disease that is two to five times that of people without the condition.

How It Happens

Just as diabetes changes the shape of the small blood vessels (known as **microvascular** changes), it also appears to thicken and obstruct the walls of the large blood vessels, thus restricting blood flow. These are called **macrovascular** changes. Macrovascular changes (such as arteriosclerosis, or hardening of the arteries) have been called the "underlying event" behind most cardiovascular disease. There's no doubt about it: Cardiovascular complications are very debilitating side effects of diabetes. However, the risk for such complications can be decreased by tight blood-sugar control.

Recognizing Risk Factors

Many factors can put a person with diabetes at risk of having a stroke or heart attack. Just having diabetes increases a person's risk of experiencing a stroke, according to the *American Journal of Epidemiology*, regardless of whether or not the person has another risk factor—for example, if he follows a sedentary lifestyle, eats a high-fat diet, has high blood pressure, or smokes cigarettes. High blood pressure alone is a major cause of strokes.

Heart attacks and strokes are more common in people with type 2 diabetes than in those with type 1 diabetes, yet medical science is not sure exactly why this is. Experts believe it could be because people with type 2 diabetes tend to be overweight. (Obesity is a known risk factor for heart attack and stroke.)

Cardiovascular complications are, in the general population, more common in men than in women: Women experience strokes and heart attacks less frequently than men. Among people *with* diabetes, however, the men and women (especially those with type 2 diabetes) have an equal chance of suffering poor outcomes after heart attacks; they have a much higher cardiovascular death rate than their nondiabetic peers.

Overall, women seem to have a biological advantage when it comes to cardiovascular disease—most likely because of the effects of estrogen in women's systems. However, diabetes appears to be the great equalizer of the sexes, at least where heart attacks are concerned. Compared with men without diabetes, men with diabetes have about two times the average risk of developing cardiovascular disease; women with diabetes have three to five times the average risk of developing cardiovascular disease compared with women without the disease.

Handling the Problem

Because the rates of cardiovascular disease are so high in those with diabetes, the American Diabetes Association recommends regular screening tests and intervention for heart disease for everyone with diabetes over age thirty.

Traditional screening tests include having your blood pressure taken with a blood pressure cuff and having your cholesterol evaluated with a blood test. An electrocardiogram (EKG) is also recommended. In this test, electrical leads are placed on the body to measure the electrical currents of the heart. The currents are then transcribed into a pattern along a continuous strip of graph paper, which is then read for any abnormalities.

To prevent heart disease in the first place, you can look to the obvious tactics of losing weight and lowering blood sugar in addition to some other methods. For example, if you've paid any attention to medical news in the past decade, then you should know that lowering levels of cholesterol and **triglycerides** is good for your heart. Cholesterol, a fatlike substance that comes from meat and diary products and is also produced by the body, is found in all the body's cells and in the bloodstream. High levels of cholesterol in the blood, or **hypercholesterolemia,** have been implicated in the development of heart disease in general and arteriosclerosis (hardening of the arteries) in particular.

What you may not know is that people with diabetes tend to have higher blood-cholesterol levels than other people. They also tend to have higher levels of **low-density lipoprotein**

(LDL), what some call the "bad cholesterol" because it aids in the deposit of fats on artery and cell walls. As if that weren't bad enough, people with diabetes tend to have lower levels of the "good cholesterol," or **high-density lipoprotein (HDL),** the substance that escorts excess cholesterol from the body. All of this is unpleasant news for the cardiovascular system.

Triglycerides (sometimes known as **VLDL,** or very-low-density lipoprotein) are another form of fat in the body. High levels of triglycerides in the blood **(hypertriglyceridemia)** may not directly cause arteriosclerosis but may accompany other abnormalities that speed its development. People with diabetes tend to have high levels of triglycerides, too. Combine high triglyceride levels of 200 to 500 mg/dl with cholesterol levels between 200 and 300 mg/dl, and you have what the *American Heart Journal* calls *combined* **hyperlipidemia,** meaning too much fat. Triglycerides more than 500 mg/dl and/or cholesterol levels over 300 mg/dl are called *massive hyperlipidemia.* Combined and massive hyperlipidemia are found in over 30 percent of all people with diabetes—approximately two to three times more often than in people without diabetes.

We talk more about cholesterol and triglycerides in the next chapter when we examine diet. For now, it's enough to say that any person with diabetes who improves his cholesterol picture can help protect against developing cardiovascular problems. Evidence suggests that for every 1 percent reduction in blood-cholesterol level, there is a 2 percent reduction in coronary-artery disease for all people, regardless of whether they have diabetes.

Another thing that people with diabetes can do to reduce their risk of cardiovascular disease is to pop a simple pill, an aspirin. The remedy was discovered because a curious thing happened during the course of a clinical study known as the Early Treatment Diabetic Retinopathy Study.

Designed to gauge the effects of aspirin on diabetic retinopathy, the study included 3,700 people with type 1 and type 2 diabetes. Half took two aspirins a day (totaling 650 milligrams); the other half took a placebo. It turned out the aspirin had no effect, positive or negative, on retinopathy. But something positive did take place: People taking aspirin were 17 percent less likely to have had a heart attack during the five years of the study.

Aspirin can't solve all the cardiovascular woes of someone with diabetes, nor is aspirin useful for everyone. But it would be worth a trip to the doctor to discuss what aspirin can do for you.

Your doctor may also suggest treatment with drugs such as beta blockers or ACE (angiotensin-converting enzyme) inhibitors—which help reduce the risk of heart attack in people who already have cardiovascular disease—or simvastatin, a drug that helps lower cholesterol levels and reduces the risk of death from heart attack.

NEUROPATHY

Neuropathy is nerve damage. The word "damage" suggests something irrevocable and permanent, but actually, this is one long-term complication of diabetes with symptoms that can appear and disappear in a short period of time. It also varies in intensity, ranging from mild discomfort to severe, disabling pain.

How It Happens

As is true about many diabetic complications, neuropathy has stumped medical science when it comes to its causes. It's thought that something interferes with the body's nerve pathways so that nerve impulses are no longer transmitted properly. The culprit may be uncontrolled blood-sugar levels (although many people with good control develop this complication), or it may be that the nerves are somehow damaged during the metabolic changes associated with diabetes.

Neuropathy is relatively common. It's estimated that some form of nerve damage affects 60 to 70 percent of people with diabetes at some point in their lives. Some physicians claim that it's often the first noticeable sign of diabetes, particularly type 2. Unfortunately, neuropathy mimics many other medical conditions (as you'll see in a moment), so it's often initially diagnosed as something else.

Recognizing the Signs

In general, there are two main forms of neuropathy: **peripheral** and **autonomic.** The most common form of nerve damage, peripheral neuropathy, is sometimes called *sensory neuropathy* because it affects nerves that control sensations in the body. It also affects muscles controlled by sensory nerves. Sensory neuropathy can weaken muscles in the thighs, eyes, chest, and abdomen, sometimes causing painful muscle wasting, double vision and chest pain. More commonly, sensory neuropathy creates odd sensations (or, in some cases, loss of sensation) in the legs, feet, and hands. The sensations include numbness, tingling, muscle weakness, and sporadic shooting pains. These sensations can be mild or they can be annoying. Some people experience double vision for short periods of time; others have great difficulty walking because of pain or because they lose some control of leg movements. Neuropathy has been known to interfere with sleep or rest.

In general, peripheral neuropathy is a temporary condition— one that disappears as mysteriously as it appears. However, it can lead to injury in cases where the person with diabetes feels no sensations of pain. This often happens on the bottoms of the feet, resulting in some of the foot problems that we discuss shortly.

Autonomic neuropathy is a less common complication, perhaps experienced by 20 percent of people with diabetes. Autonomic neuropathy is damage to the nerves that control various bodily functions, such as the digestive system, urinary tract, and cardiovascular system.

Autonomic neuropathy leads to many inconvenient problems: When it affects the nerves around the stomach, bladder, and bowels, it can cause vomiting, constipation, and feelings of bloatedness. When it affects the nerves that control the contraction of blood vessels, a condition called **orthostatic hypotension** may develop. This is a sudden drop in blood pressure when a person gets up after reclining, which may result in dizziness or fainting. **Impotence,** the loss of the ability to have an erection, is also related to (although not entirely caused by) neuropathic damage.

Handling the Problem

The symptoms of neuropathy of both types can be treated. Doctors often prescribe drugs to treat the symptoms of these different problems—for example, to relax muscles if the problem is constipation. Exercise helps some people; others benefit from bed rest. Because neuropathy varies tremendously from person to person, treating it is often a matter of trial and error.

But though symptoms can be treated, neuropathy itself cannot be reversed. Medications to treat or prevent nerve damage do not yet exist, although researchers are conducting studies using aldose reductase inhibitors—experimental drugs we discussed earlier in relation to retinopathy.

FOOT PROBLEMS

Cardiovascular complications damage blood vessels and diminish blood flow to the legs and feet. Add damage to the nerves of the legs and feet through neuropathy, and you've just laid the groundwork for serious foot ailments.

How They Happen

Foot ailments show up in about half of people who have had diabetes for 20 years or more. The scenario then proceeds like this: When people with diabetes lose sensation in their lower legs and feet, they are less likely to notice damage to the skin and tissues. Such seemingly minor injuries as cuts, bruises, blisters, bunions, corns, calluses, ingrown toenails, or even athlete's foot can develop into areas of infected tissue known as **neuropathic ulcers.**

It may seem impossible that a blister turns into an ulcer, yet the process is fairly simple. Let's say you have a new pair of shoes that has chafed and rubbed one foot raw. The area is red and inflamed. Once an inflammation or infection begins, its swelling compresses the blood vessels, which are already damaged or narrowed by diabetes itself. These factors diminish the flow of blood to the irritated area, meaning fresh oxygen and infection-fighting blood cells have a more difficult time getting to the problem site.

All of this sets the stage for a serious infection. Once infection sets in, it's difficult to treat. Antibiotics, which are carried in the blood, can't reach the infected area efficiently. About 80 percent of foot ulcers occur on the bottom of insensate feet, or feet without feeling.

The real danger with the combination of infection and reduced blood flow is **gangrene.** If blood flow were to be completely blocked, the cells served by the obstructed blood vessels would die. Once gangrene sets in, the only way to stop its spread is by amputation of the dead tissue.

According to an article in *Archives of Internal Medicine,* "It has been estimated that the lifetime risk of a lower-extremity amputation is 5 to 15 percent among diabetic individuals, a risk fifteen times that of the nondiabetic population."

More than half of all lower-limb amputations in the United States are performed on people with diabetes. Each year, reports the American Podiatric Medical Association, the number of lower-limb amputations due to diabetic complications in the United States exceeds the number of limbs lost worldwide to land mines. Almost half of these 67,000 amputations could have been prevented through early detection and treatment.

Recognizing Risk Factors

As is true with all diabetic complications, certain factors increase risk of foot problems. The greatest of these is smoking. According to the American Diabetes Association, of the people with diabetes who need amputations, almost all are smokers. Other high-risk factors include being male and being African-American or Native American. Risk increases with age, too.

A 1998 study published in the *Archives of Internal Medicine* listed a number of criteria doctors can use to determine a patient's risk of foot ulcers. These include a history of amputation, diabetes for more than ten years, existing foot deformities, neuropathy, and difficulty feeling vibrations with the feet. The study authors encouraged practitioners to survey for these criteria in order to prevent such complications.

Handling the Problem

The trick to treating and preventing foot problems lies in finding out if a blood vessel is about to become blocked. It used to be that doctors could locate blockages in large vessels, such as those of the legs, only by ordering an x-ray called an **angiogram.** Then they might perform **bypass surgery** to detour blood around the blockage. In this surgery, a piece of healthy vein is "harvested" from an area of the body (possibly the thigh) and is attached at either end of the obstruction. The new vein directs blood to cells that had been receiving an inadequate supply. It's one method of preventing gangrene—albeit an invasive and expensive one.

There is now another way to prevent foot ulcers, gangrene, and amputation. A simple low-tech test can prevent at least 27,000 amputations of toes and feet a year (half the current annual total), according to the Lower Extremity Amputation Prevention (LEAP) program sponsored by the U.S. Department of Health and Human Services (HHS).

The painless test is performed using a **monofilament,** a long, flexible nylon bristle. By pressing this calibrated nylon filament against each of ten predetermined places on the foot, your health care practitioner can determine whether you are losing sensation in your foot. If you are, you and your practitioner can take steps to keep foot ulcers from developing. And the test is (or should be) inexpensive: The reusable monofilaments are available for as little as $10 each. A monofilament test that people with diabetes can perform themselves is also being developed to serve as an adjunct to a test by a physician.

Researchers have also come up with a gel that improves the healing of diabetic ulcers. The becaplermin gel, called Regranex, was approved in 1998 by FDA. The gel contains a growth factor that stimulates healing, making it the first prescription drug to actually stimulate the body to grow new tissue and heal a wound.

Like many other diabetic complications we discuss in this chapter, amputation doesn't have to happen. With proper foot care, many, if not most, amputations may well be avoided.

CHAPTER FIVE

Self-Care: Putting Yourself in Control

As you have learned, diabetes is a complicated disease. But self-care really can make a difference in how the disease affects you. Unlike many other illnesses, *most of the control of diabetes rests in the hands of the patient.* Self-care is not just important, it's absolutely essential.

This chapter (and indeed, this entire book) is designed to help people with diabetes take charge of their own treatment to the best of their ability. Keep in mind that the overall goal of any treatment is to control blood sugar—to keep it within normal limits. Working toward that goal entails reevaluating your lifestyle, adopting a new meal plan and a regular exercise routine, and making a commitment to self-monitoring of blood glucose. It also entails being aware of the symptoms and dangers of the potential complications of diabetes—those problems discussed in Chapter 4.

The responsibility may seem overwhelming, and it may be difficult to tell where to begin. If you have type 1 diabetes, you need to understand the ways in which insulin, food, and exercise affect blood sugar. Insulin we discussed in depth in Chapter 2; food and exercise are addressed in this chapter.

If you have type 2 diabetes, you need to understand the role of obesity, exercise, and food consumption in insulin resistance. You may have to lose weight and become physically active. These latter two things are more than a matter of looking good—they're about making it easier for your body to produce and use insulin.

There's no easy way around all of this. The fact of the matter remains: Managing your diabetes is demanding and, at times, difficult. It's a daily, lifelong process. And even when you try your best, your condition can still get out of hand. But the alternative—neglecting the disease—poses such demonstrated drawbacks that most folks opt for self-care.

Self-Monitoring of Blood Glucose

As was mentioned at the start of this book, the real goal is to control your diabetes instead of letting it control you. And the encouraging news is that control is literally in your hands! Self-monitoring of blood glucose, or SMBG, is a hands-on method of tracking blood sugar. With SMBG, you can test your blood-sugar level at home, in the office, on the road—any place and any time, as often as you wish. It gives people with diabetes a new level of flexibility—they don't have to make a trip to a doctor's office whenever they want an accurate blood-glucose reading, as was the case years ago.

Because SMBG can provide the information needed to balance food intake, exercise, and insulin or medication, it has rapidly become a mainstay of diabetes-management plans. Doctors aren't always keen on consumer self-care and self-testing, but the health care profession as a whole has embraced self-monitoring of blood glucose. It may well be the best invention for people with diabetes since the discovery of insulin.

Performing SMBG is far from difficult, though it's not quite pleasant. Using a special needle called a **lancet,** a person with diabetes pricks his finger and then places a drop of blood either on a test strip or on a specially treated sensor pad on a glucose meter, a device about the size of a hand calculator. Some test strips change color depending upon the amount of glucose in the blood, and the color is compared with a master chart. Other strips are inserted into a glucose meter, and one recently approved monitor uses cartridges of test strips for the sake of convenience. The blood-glucose meter indicates just how many milligrams of glucose are present in a decaliter of blood. The reading appears on the meter's display panel in numbers, and the whole test is complete within minutes.

Self-monitoring is valuable for anyone who is at all concerned about managing diabetes. Because the process is relatively quick, it can be done many times a day, giving the person

On the Horizon

Daily finger sticks are not exactly fun. Fortunately, researchers are busy creating noninvasive devices for blood-glucose monitoring with the hope that such devices will take away the discomfort of needles. And if such devices encourage people with diabetes to test their blood sugar levels more often, there are direct benefits to a diabetic person's health.

One such noninvasive blood-glucose monitor—a work in progress—is a device that uses infrared light to measure the amount of glucose in the blood. This "dream beam" is based on the fact that every substance has a unique optical signature—glucose included—when viewed with infrared light. The device sends a beam of light (which can't be seen or felt) that penetrates the skin and identifies glucose by its optical signature. The amount of glucose is then calculated by the device and displayed as a reading—without any blood being shed. One such meter was already submitted to the U.S. Food and Drug Administration (FDA) for review—and rejected—but similar devices may soon be presented for approval.

Also in the works is a patch that would draw interstitial fluid (the fluid that surrounds cells) through the skin. The patch reacts to the glucose in the fluid, and the reaction is monitored and translated into a blood-glucose measurement by a separate device worn on the wrist like a watch. This device, called the GlucoWatch system, is under review by FDA as this book goes to press.

In late 1998, FDA approved the Lasette, laser finger perforator that allows drawing of blood in a nearly painless manner for glucose testing. The Lasette—the first laser-based medical device ever cleared by FDA for home use—offers people a means of drawing blood without using traditional lancets. Research has found that diabetic people who are adequately trained in the use of the device can test themselves as easily and accurately as with lancets. Further, according to one researcher, many people experience far less pain using the Lasette, and their fingers appear to heal faster.

a clear picture of how his blood glucose fluctuates throughout the day. When blood sugar slides outside of target levels, the person can take action.

SMBG: WHO NEEDS IT?

These days self-monitoring is recommended for anyone who uses insulin—whether the person has type 1, type 2, or gestational diabetes. Many doctors insist that adjustments in insulin doses should be based on blood-glucose measurements. One reason is that even an identical dose of insulin will be absorbed differently from day to day, depending on factors such as insulin sensitivity, exercise, stress, types of food eaten, and hormonal changes (puberty, the menstrual cycle, and pregnancy, for example).

Self-monitoring is also suggested when someone begins insulin therapy or changes to a new insulin species, brand, or dose. (See Chapter 2 for a review of insulin terms.) During the adjustment or transition period, people with diabetes use SMBG to carefully track blood-glucose levels and ensure they are within target ranges.

SMBG is also a good idea for those people with type 2 diabetes who are using oral hypoglycemic agents, because those folks face the danger of very low blood sugar when using those drugs.

Further, there are circumstances in which doctors say SMBG is mandatory. SMBG is required for people who are following a tight-control regimen, whether via insulin pump, frequent insulin injections, oral hypoglycemic agents, or combination therapy. As we discussed in Chapters 2 and 4, people following a tight-control regimen are more able to keep their blood-sugar levels on a near-normal even keel, but they are prone to frequent bouts of hypoglycemia, or dangerously low blood sugar.

Frequent self-monitoring can flag falling blood-sugar levels before they become disruptive.

Another circumstance that calls for mandatory SMBG is illness, sometimes referred to as physical stress. Illness wreaks havoc with the body's blood-sugar levels, often increasing sugar even if someone does not eat or drink. Thus, people with diabetes generally need to take more insulin when they are sick. But how much more? The results of self-monitoring can guide them and their doctors in making that decision. In fact, in any case where they are forced to step off their regular medication plans and wander into uncharted territory, SMBG is essential—a compass in the wilderness.

Certain other circumstances necessitate monitoring of blood glucose. People who have wide swings in blood-sugar levels often turn to SMBG to find out why. You may have heard of the term **brittle diabetes;** it describes a rare condition, generally found only among people with type 1 diabetes, in which blood-sugar levels fluctuate dramatically from day to day.

The wide swings of brittle diabetes may be caused by poor management of the disease. Or they may have at their root a completely different hormonal disorder, another disease, or the side effects of drugs. At any rate, self-monitoring can help someone with diabetes track sugar swings and determine how much insulin is necessary, depending upon each day's blood-sugar levels.

Beyond SMBG

If blood-glucose levels fall too low, another self-care test, the urine-ketone test (also known as the urine-acetone test because ketones are sometimes called acetones) comes into play. It detects the presence of ketones, or toxins, in the blood. Ketones are formed when fat instead of glucose is burned for energy, which happens when there is no insulin in the blood. People with type 1 diabetes use the urine-ketone test when their blood-sugar levels are low to check for the life-threatening condition ketoacidosis, or diabetic coma, which we talk about in Chapter 2.

As we mentioned earlier, SMBG is growing in standing with the medical profession. Your doctor may proffer other reasons to practice this simple self-care technique.

PUTTING SMBG TO WORK

How often SMBG is performed should be determined by the patient and the doctor, although most would agree that haphazard or infrequent measurement—say, only once a week—can give little information to go on.

That said, there are some commonly recommended measurement patterns. For instance, people just beginning SMBG may be instructed to check their blood sugar four to eight times a day, including first thing in the morning, before and after each meal, and last thing before bed.

People using insulin (including people with type 1 and type 2 diabetes) may average four checks a day: before each meal and late in the evening.

People with type 2 diabetes who have their sugar under control have the greatest flexibility. Their monitoring schedule might include a morning check four to seven times a week along with the occasional before-meal or bedtime test.

As we imply, people with diabetes generally test their blood before meals. Those who use insulin need these readings to determine how much insulin to take. Some folks like to take the occasional reading after a meal (known as a **postprandial** reading) because that's the time when blood sugar shoots up. It can help to gauge how high sugar goes after food consumption.

At certain times, blood sugar should be monitored more frequently than usual. These situations include illness, changes in medication, travel, or any change in routine. Basically any change in lifestyle, including a new job, a new exercise pattern, a different diet (one that may occur when visiting friends or relatives, for example), relocation, a job change, marriage, or retirement may cause changes in blood-sugar levels. Travel through several time zones, especially by air, makes it more difficult to time medications and meals. Here, SMBG can give people with diabetes the information they need for dose adjustments. (Doctors can give special advice about insulin administration when traveling great distances, such as overseas. Self-monitoring will still be important, though.)

In addition, someone can voluntarily increase the frequency of monitoring whenever he wants more information about what's happening in his body. SMBG is primarily used for adjusting insulin doses. In the short term, self-monitoring tells you what action you need to take to get blood sugar within the target range set by you and your doctor. But SMBG is also used to build a larger picture—a month-by-month, year-by-year image of what doctors call **glycemic control,** or overall control of blood-sugar levels.

SMBG enables people with diabetes to build a database of sorts. Toward this end, many start a notebook, diary, or computerized record and write down the results of their blood-glucose tests. (Some of the new blood-glucose meters store this information in an electronic memory.) Over time, these details disclose how their blood sugar reacts to exercise, to certain foods, to travel, and to other environmental factors. With information in hand, people then discuss results with their doctors during routine office visits. Ultimately, all of these pieces of information help fine-tune the diabetes management program.

Another benefit of getting to know what's normal for your body is being able to spot a developing problem or emergency, such as an unusually high (or unusually low) blood-glucose reading.

The Cost of Monitoring

Clearly, blood-sugar monitoring four times a day can be valuable to your health, but it may also take its toll on your pocketbook. People with diabetes spend somewhere in the neighborhood of $396 million each year on blood-glucose-measuring devices alone, according to one estimate. And the market for these devices is growing.

The cost of meters and supplies averages $1,000 a year for someone using an SMBG monitor. Part of the price depends on your choice of equipment—necessities such as lancets, test strips, and glucose meters. Many of today's high-tech glucose meters have sticker prices of $50, $150, and up. Some manufacturers offer meters at steep discounts, knowing that consumers must purchase test strips or other supplies specifically developed for those meters.

New versions of blood-glucose kits arrive on the market every season. The trend is toward developing new products that make self-testing simpler, more convenient, and quicker. Blood-glucose meters, for example, have become smaller and less cumbersome in recent years—good news if you're inclined to tote a meter along with you on your daily travels.

In actuality, SMBG is a small part of the total cost of diabetes care. But add in the cost of blood tests performed in a doctor's office (we discuss those later in this chapter), and the annual tab for blood monitoring can easily exceed $1,600—which may be covered by many (but not all) health insurers. Yet if self-monitoring delays or prevents the pain, the aggravation, and the cost of diabetic complications, then that money is well spent.

THE ACCURACY OF SMBG

If you've been in the market for a monitoring system, you may have noticed the use of the words "error rate" and "error range" on labels and in literature, suggesting that blood-glucose meters aren't accurate. And many of them are not. In fact, one study from the College of American Pathologists found meter readings off by as much as 33 percent in some systems it tested.

Some amount of error is acceptable. According to an American Diabetes Association (ADA) consensus statement, all SMBG systems should strive for the goal of an error rate of less than 10 percent. Translated, that means blood-glucose readings from meters can be off by as much as 10 percent and still be valuable. At first blush, it seems like a large number. But experts view SMBG as more accurate than the urine-sugar test, which was previously the only sugar test people could perform at home (and an imprecise one at that).

The error rate of glucose meters can be caused by many things. Sometimes it's a matter of improper technique with the lancet or the meter itself. Mishandling the meter (such as dropping it or leaving it in a hot car) can cause it to malfunction. Improper storage of test strips (exposing them to intense sun or moisture) can lead to a faulty reading.

Easing the Burden

Keeping diabetes in check can be expensive, what with the cost of glucose monitors, test strips, lancets, medications, insulin, and syringes. And unfortunately, in the face of such costs, some people with diabetes cut corners on their care to save some money—perhaps by performing SMBG less often.

A 1997 Gallup poll of 250 large employers found that many did not cover basic laboratory tests, blood glucose monitors, or education programs for those with diabetes under their insurance programs. However, in July 1998, the federal government began a new Medicare reimbursement program that covers the cost of glucose test strips and monitors for all beneficiaries with diabetes. The plan also pays for education for diabetes patients on an outpatient basis; previously, such classes were covered only if they took place in the hospital. In addition, $300 million will be provided for diabetes research and grants over the next five years. Medications and insulin still are not covered.

It is hoped the change will encourage and enable those with diabetes to monitor their conditions more closely—and not just because the government is concerned about a person's health. The fact is that some $318 billion each year is spent on diabetes, with complications such as blindness, cardiovascular disease, and neuropathy accounting for most of those costs. By offering monitoring and education, the government hopes to prevent these expensive and often disabling complications.

Another chunk of the blame for misreadings and errors can be put on the quality of instruction that people receive. In 1991, a warning was delivered by an advocacy panel of health professionals, consumers, researchers, and manufacturers known as the National Steering Committee for Quality Assurance in Capillary Blood Glucose Monitoring. The committee's research found that "many monitoring errors result from improper training, misunderstanding of instructional materials and bad habits developed over long periods of unsupervised self-monitoring." The panel "implored" physicians, meter manufacturers, and other health care professionals "to improve the way self-monitoring is taught and evaluated," in the words of the report.

Today, blood-glucose monitoring has been made somewhat easier through technological advancement, but patient education still plays an important role. After all, if self-testing is done incorrectly, the results could be way off. The American Diabetes Association stresses that health care providers teach their patients how to use SMBG. They recommend providers ask people to demonstrate their testing techniques and then compare the results with laboratory tests of blood glucose. This way, a practitioner can determine if a person is testing himself correctly and whether his equipment is calibrated accurately.

Accuracy of blood tests is important to all people with diabetes, but particularly to those who follow the insulin therapy regimen of tight control we discuss in Chapter 2. That's because those folks have a two to three times greater risk of developing hypoglycemia—dangerously low blood-sugar levels—than people on conventional insulin therapy. Some experts postulate that incorrect insulin dosing as a result of monitoring errors may be one reason hypoglycemia is so common.

The message here for all people who practice self-monitoring is clear: Be an informed consumer! Get one-on-one training in meter use, perhaps from two or more people. Ask questions if you get conflicting or inconsistent advice.

Nutrition and Diabetes

Whatever the form, self-testing is only one player on the diabetes self-care team. Another major player is nutrition—the foods we eat.

Because diabetes is basically a misfunction in the body's ability to use food as energy, food is an important part of the treatment plan. The kinds of foods a person with diabetes eats, for example, will influence the course of the disease.

No two ways about it: Diet, or the eating plan, as it is known, is crucial in the treatment and management of diabetes. That's why people first diagnosed with diabetes are often referred to a dietitian for assistance in analyzing their eating habits and forging better eating plans.

A new eating plan may mean major changes in the way you eat. It will be necessary to eat well, following sound nutritional principles. You'll have to make some adjustments, perhaps in how much you eat, perhaps in how often, perhaps in what you eat. Whether or not this is a major change depends upon how you've been eating in the past—something we can't tell from where we're sitting.

The *Joslin Diabetes Manual* neatly summarizes the situation: "While some people with diabetes do have to make major diet restrictions, what most lose is the right to overeat or make poor food choices."

GETTING INTO GUIDELINES

So what are the proper food choices? Evidence from many recent studies documents the importance of a high-fiber, high-complex-carbohydrate diet in improving glucose metabolism. This is a relatively recent change—one that began in 1979 and continued into the mid-1980s as the American Diabetes Association revised its nutritional guidelines to reflect changing research findings. Before then, doctors had always steered their patients toward a low-carbohydrate diet.

As you know, food consists of three nutrients: proteins, fats, and carbohydrates. Proteins are used to refurbish the body, replacing worn-out cells with vigorous new ones. Fats are a semi-permanent form of nutrient storage. You might envision them as an emergency or backup fuel system.

But when it comes to keeping the body running (or walking or talking), carbohydrates are the real workhorses of the nutrient family. During digestion, carbohydrates are converted either into glucose or glycogen. Glucose is used for immediate energy. Glycogen is glucose in temporary storage, poised and ready to be retrieved at precisely the moment the body calls for energy.

The American Diabetes Association's nutritional guidelines suggest that you should work with your health care team to determine your diet: No diet is appropriate for all people. The ADA does offer some rough guidelines, however. Proteins should account for only 10 to 20 percent of total calories (an even lower amount is suggested for some people with diabetic nephropathy, a form of kidney disease that we discussed in Chapter 4). Fewer than 30 percent of calories should come from fat, with saturated and polyunsaturated fats each accounting for fewer than 10 percent. For fiber, the recommendation is 20 to 35 grams of fiber daily.

Because carbohydrates can have a great effect on blood-sugar levels, the ADA says that the percentage of calories from carbohydrates eaten daily should depend upon the individual, and it refrains from making a specific recommendation. However, previous recommendations were in the 55 to 60 percent range.

The diet recommended for those with diabetes isn't much different than one someone without the condition should follow. This "diabetic diet" is the same eating plan that is now recommended for the U.S. population in general. For people

Differences in Diets

While the diet recommended by the American Diabetes Association is well established, research is afoot to reexamine, through clinical studies, the type 2 diabetic diet. These researchers are testing a nutritional plan called the 40 percent-40 percent diet, an experimental plan for type 2 diabetes that reduces saturated fat intake. Under this plan, 40 percent of total calories come from monounsaturated fats (such as olive oil and canola oil—fats that may have a heart-healthy effect) and 40 percent from carbohydrates. Researchers think that large amounts of carbohydrates increase triglyceride levels in poorly controlled type 2 diabetes.

Another diet, this one low in carbohydrates, has been devised by Richard K. Bernstein, M.D., in his book *Diabetes Type II* (New York: Prentice Hall, 1990). He recommends that people with type 2 diabetes eat only 30 grams of carbohydrates a day—equivalent to 2 1/2 slices of bread.

Bernstein argues that a high-carbohydrate meal makes it impossible to attain normal blood-sugar levels for several hours after eating, and he strives to keep blood-sugar levels normal at all points in the day. (In contrast, most doctors expect and accept a higher postprandial, or after-meal, blood-sugar reading.)

Under Bernstein's plan, verboten foods include simple sugars, cereals, bread and flour products, rice, certain cooked vegetables (carrots, potatoes, corn, beets, and tomatoes), and just about all foods found on the shelves of the average health food store. His approved foods include most vegetables; meat, fish, fowl, and eggs; most cheeses; nuts; and soy products.

If you have type 2 diabetes and have difficulty digesting high-fiber carbohydrates, or if a high-fiber, high-carbohydrate diet doesn't seem to control your blood sugar, then you might wish to consider a low-carbohydrate diet.

These conflicting opinions are very disorienting for those trying to decide on a treatment. However, you can't make the decision alone. It's always essential for people with diabetes, as medical consumers, to delve into issues and discuss them with their doctor. The moral is: Speak up!

with diabetes with a family, this is good news: It means a healthy diabetic meal for them is one that the rest of the family can share.

People with type 1 and type 2 diabetes do not need to eat foods different from each other, either. As we said, the basic nutritional principles apply to all, so the foods remain the same. However, the goals of diet therapy differ.

People with type 1 diabetes follow a simple formula: Eating increases blood sugar; exercise and insulin lower blood sugar. For that reason, people with type 1 diabetes are very concerned with the timing of their meals. Meals and snacks must be coordinated with insulin injections and exercise so that blood sugar always remains within target levels.

People with type 2 diabetes must remember that eating increases blood sugar and that consuming a lot of calories at one time can overwhelm the body's limited ability to use insulin efficiently. This limited ability, or insulin resistance, seems to be triggered or intensified by obesity. Since most people with type 2 diabetes are overweight, their diet goals center on reducing food consumption (which reduces insulin demands on the body) and losing weight (which enables what insulin is present to operate more efficiently).

Since food intake affects blood glucose, both people with type 1 and people with type 2 diabetes should take care not to make any major changes in their diets without consulting their physicians. To help you understand a little more about how diets are put together, here's a rundown of some of the most important nutritional players and their relationship with diabetes.

Fat

Fats are a problem for most Americans, not just people with diabetes. High levels of dietary fat have been shown to increase the risk of cardiovascular disease primarily through the effects of fats (known as cholesterol and triglycerides) in the blood.

On top of this, fat is just plain fattening! One gram of fat contains nine calories, but one gram of protein or carbohydrate contains only four calories. Since many people with diabetes are overweight, reducing fat consumption is the quickest way to begin cutting calories.

Fat comes in three forms—saturated, polyunsaturated, and monounsaturated. Generally, people are encouraged to eat some of all three, but to minimize saturated fat.

To understand why that is, let's look at where fats are found:

Saturated fats come from meat and dairy products, although certain tropical oils (cocoa butter and coconut, palm, and palm-kernel oils) are also highly saturated.

Polyunsaturated fats come from vegetable oils, including corn, cottonseed, safflower, soybean, and sunflower.

Monounsaturated fats are found in olive and canola oils and in avocados.

Both polyunsaturated and monounsaturated fats are liquid at room temperature. They also appear to lower cholesterol when they replace saturated fats in the diet, namely because saturated fats encourage the body to produce more cholesterol. Cutting out the saturated fats helps cholesterol levels to drop. And lowering cholesterol is a good thing, especially for people with diabetes.

Cholesterol

Years ago, diabetes management simply revolved around glycemic control. Now physicians know that control of fats, or lipid levels, in the blood is just as important. This is because a high cholesterol level is a major risk factor for heart disease

Type of Fat May Combat Diabetes

Fat has long been the enemy in the war against diabetes. However, researchers have begun preliminary studies of a fat that may help prevent diabetes.

The fat, known as conjugated linoleic acid (CLA), is found in red meats and cheese. It is thought to work like diabetes drugs in the thiazolidinedione class, which help sensitize the body to insulin. (Troglitazone, which we talk about in Chapter 3, is a thiazolidinedione.) In studies from Purdue University and Pennsylvania State University in 1998, researchers found that rats that were bred to develop diabetes did not get the disease when they were fed the fats.

Further research—including human trials—is planned for CLA. Researchers hope the fat could lead to new drugs or dietary strategies for those with diabetes.

and atherosclerosis (a build up of plaque blockages within the arteries). And as we said in Chapter 4, people with diabetes are more likely to develop high cholesterol levels.

For reasons yet unknown, high blood sugar tends to increase cholesterol levels in the blood. Therefore, both type 1 and type 2 diabetes cause higher cholesterol levels if blood-sugar levels are poorly controlled. For example, extremely high levels of triglycerides (a form of fat that contributes to the development of arteriosclerosis, or hardening of the arteries) are commonly found in people experiencing diabetic ketoacidosis.

What's more, lowering blood sugar can lower cholesterol and triglycerides. It appears that the key to low levels of LDL cholesterol (the bad cholesterol) and triglycerides and high levels of HDL (the good cholesterol) lies in glycemic control. In a nutshell, that means carefully managing your disease by using an eating plan, insulin or oral agent, weight loss, exercise, or (most likely) some combination of these.

Reducing your cholesterol is important. If you already have high LDL and triglyceride levels, your risk for heart disease increases with each additional lifestyle risk, such as obesity, inactivity, high blood pressure, and tobacco use. That's because high fat levels, arterial-wall changes, insulin levels, hypertension, and obesity are all factors that combine to accelerate arteriosclerosis in people with diabetes.

Because high cholesterol is so dangerous, the ADA recommends changing your diet to lower cholesterol and reduce the risk of heart disease. Evidence suggests that for every 1 percent reduction in blood-cholesterol level, there is a 2 percent reduction in coronary-artery disease. In addition, the ADA recommends drug therapy to lower high cholesterol in patients who have heart disease.

Even **total serum cholesterol** levels (the overall amount of cholesterol in the blood) and LDL-cholesterol levels that are considered borderline for nondiabetic persons are probably of concern in those with diabetes.

As usual, specific goals of which levels to try for vary from person to person; your doctor can help you set precise parameters. But to give you a snapshot of what works for some, here's a list of management goals set by the University of Kentucky Metabolic Research Group in Lexington for its adult patients:

- Total serum cholesterol: less than 200 mg/dl

- Fasting serum triglycerides: less than 250 mg/d

- LDL cholesterol: less than 130 mg/dl

- HDL cholesterol: over 45 mg/dl in men, over 55 mg/dl in women

- Reaching desirable body weight

Carbohydrates

One way to lower your cholesterol levels is to remove the source of cholesterol in your diet by replacing foods high in saturated fats with fiber-rich carbohydrates. According to the American Diabetes Association, a person with diabetes should work with a physician to determine the percent of daily calories that should be derived from complex carbohydrates.

Carbohydrates come in two forms: simple and complex. Simple carbohydrates can be quickly converted into glucose. They also cause a swift rise in blood-glucose levels. Simple carbohydrates are often called simple sugars. They include soft drinks, candy, and sugars (table or granulated sugar, brown sugar, molasses, and so forth).

Many people believe that complex carbohydrates are better for those with diabetes than simple sugars. However, there's little scientific evidence to support that belief. As a result, there's no reason to eliminate sugar from your diet if you're concerned about your blood-sugar levels. For many people this may come as a surprise: Sugar (in moderation) is not taboo. Today's research shows that sugar intake by itself doesn't govern blood-glucose levels. For example, one recent study found that people with type 1 diabetes could eat two sugar-laden snacks a day (snacks such as brownies and ice cream) with no effect on glycemic control! And the American Diabetes Association has given the thumbs-up on a teaspoon of sugar, honey, molasses, or other sweetener per food serving. That's twice the amount of sugar once recommended.

Artificial sweeteners are OK to use as well. Saccharin and aspartame are valid substitutes for sugar. Unlike sugar, saccharin is calorie free. Aspartame contains so few calories per serving that no one counts them.

So as you see, simple carbohydrates, or simple sugars, can have a place in a meal plan, as long as the person with diabetes realizes that sugar offers only empty calories—not exactly helpful if he is trying to lose weight. Nor is sugar recommended if the person's diabetes is not well controlled.

This brings us to complex carbohydrates. Because their cellular structure is more complex, these carbohydrates take longer to be broken down into glucose and absorbed into the bloodstream. Thus, complex carbohydrates don't increase blood-sugar levels as rapidly as simple carbohydrates. Complex carbohydrates include legumes (such as beans and peas), grains (such as rice), bread, pasta, fruits, and starchy vegetables.

Fiber

The best complex carbohydrates, according to recent research, are those that contain a lot of fiber. Fiber is the indigestible material in grains, vegetables, and fruits. Fiber can slow the speed at which carbohydrates are absorbed and converted into blood glucose.

The recommendation is that people with diabetes increase their consumption of fiber to 20 to 35 grams every day. Unfortunately, the average American eats only 11 to 23 grams of fiber daily—meaning that some folks need to double or triple their fiber consumption.

Fiber comes in two forms: insoluble and soluble. The difference between the two is pretty simple. As its name implies, insoluble fiber doesn't dissolve in water. It does absorb water, though, and helps escort foods more quickly through the intestinal system. Foods that contain insoluble fiber include wheat bran, such as that found in whole-grain breads, and certain vegetables and fruits (particularly apple skin, raw carrots, and beets).

In contrast, soluble fiber dissolves in water, turning into a thick, gelatinous mass that slows down the rate of glucose absorption. Soluble fiber is helpful for people with diabetes because it helps prevent a sharp rise in blood sugar immediately after eating. Foods high in soluble fiber include oat bran, legumes (such as navy, lima, and kidney beans), corn, apples, and oranges.

The general recommendation is that fiber intake should be increased gradually, perhaps by adding one fiber-rich food per week and including a fiber in every meal to give the body time to adapt and prevent excessive gas production, a common side effect of added fiber.

As we mentioned, fiber slows the speed at which carbohydrates are converted into glucose. And when people with diabetes increase fiber-rich foods and decrease fat-laden ones, they can reduce cholesterol levels and triglyceride levels, at least according to the results of studies at the University of Kentucky. In these studies, people with diabetes followed a diet of 55 to 60 percent carbohydrates and 25 grams of fiber per 1,000 calories. Blood cholesterol fell 1 to 20 percent and triglycerides dipped 40 percent. Researchers believe that such results clinch the argument on the value of high-fiber, high-carbohydrate eating plans.

Just as a healthy diet lowers blood sugar, it lowers insulin requirements. People with diabetes may be able to decrease their insulin doses about 10 percent; people with type 2 may be able to reduce the dose of any oral agent by one-third to one-half. And because high-fiber foods are very filling and low in fat, they can help people lose weight.

SIZING UP YOUR MEALS

Once you and your doctor figure out the right balance of protein, fat, carbohydrates, and fiber, the next step is deciding how much to eat. This is crucial for people with type 1 diabetes because the projected size of their meals determines insulin doses. Once insulin is injected, people with diabetes can't eat more or less than planned without throwing blood sugar out of whack.

Careful control of diet is also important for those with type 2 diabetes. As you may recall, part of the treatment of type 2 is reducing food intake—eating less, in effect. The reason is simple: The more food you eat, the greater the demand for insulin. Further, the amount you need to eat depends upon your age, gender, height, and the amount of exercise you get. Your health care practitioner or a dietitian can help you map out the appropriate number of calories you need each day.

Whether you have type 1 or type 2, you need to be precise about your calorie needs if you must lose weight or if you are concerned about gaining it, because too much food causes too many pounds. As the *Joslin Diabetes Manual* explains, "Obese people often look for excuses beyond their control, such as a 'glandular condition' or 'stress,' but the basic reason that they are overweight is that they have eaten more calories than they need."

People with diabetes also need to monitor the frequency of meals. Generally, the experts agree that "small feedings"—three or four small meals a day—are better than one large daily meal.

Doctors recommend that people using insulin schedule their meals so that they eat something—if only a snack—at peak insulin times. People with type 2 diabetes who don't use insulin are encouraged to spread out their caloric consumption into three meals and several snacks so that they aren't calling on their pancreas to produce large amounts of insulin to cope with one or two large meals.

And an article in the *New England Journal of Medicine* suggests another reason for spreading out caloric consumption: People who eat frequent small meals (particularly those high in soluble fiber, which prolongs absorption time) may be less likely to experience those higher levels of cholesterol and triglycerides that accompany diabetes.

THE GLYCEMIC INDEX

Once you've got a handle on the components of a balanced diet and how often to eat, you need to think specifically about the kinds of foods you're eating. You see, not all complex carbohydrates slow increases in blood glucose. As studies were done on various foods and their effects on blood sugar, researchers discovered that different carbohydrates break down at different rates. The carbohydrates in a potato, for instance, are converted into glucose more quickly than those in rice.

From this observation about the differing effect of food on blood-glucose levels came a rather controversial concept called the **glycemic index.** The glycemic index was developed by scientists at the University of Toronto to calculate how foods affect blood-glucose levels. For example, in a laboratory setting, both honey and cooked carrots raised blood-sugar levels 80 to 90 percent as high as straight glucose did, while lentils and kidney beans raised blood sugar a mere 20 to 29 percent as high as glucose did. Taking this data, scientists assigned a different glycemic value to a whole host of foods. The glycemic index was useful in scientific measurements, and the hope was that it might be useful to people with diabetes—the idea being that by knowing the glycemic value of certain foods, people would eat those foods less likely to raise blood glucose.

Although the glycemic index seems useful, it is controversial because in real life, a food's glycemic index is not a fixed number. It changes depending on whether the food is cooked, how it's cooked, how long it's cooked, and what other foods are eaten along with it. For that reason and others, experts don't see the glycemic index as a helpful tool for day-to-day meal planning.

To help people with diabetes wade through the meal-planning waters, the American Diabetes Association and the American

Dietetic Association developed the exchange system. Here's how it works: Under this system, foods are grouped into six categories: bread and starch, vegetables, fruit, milk, meat, and fat. The foods in each category, when eaten in the portions indicated, have the same number of calories and the same nutritional value. For instance, under the bread and starch category, one-third of a cup of vegetarian baked beans has the same number of calories as one slice of raisin bread.

You can see how this makes calorie counting and meal planning less painful—all the calorie-counting footwork has been done. The exchange system helps people accurately coordinate their insulin doses with the amount of food they eat. It also helps other people set up a plan to lose weight. As long as they use the specified portions, people can exchange one food under a heading with another food from that same group, knowing that both foods have the same number of calories and the same nutritional content. Information on the exchange system is available from the American Diabetes Association, the American Dietetic Association, and dietitians and physicians.

CAFFEINE AND ALCOHOL

Experts have gone back and forth recently on the risks and benefits of the daily cup of java, arriving at the conclusion that for healthy people, moderate amounts of caffeine are fine. There is also an official stand on the use of caffeine for those with diabetes. The amount of caffeine in a couple of cups of coffee or tea or in several soft drinks isn't going to affect diabetes control. For that reason, most doctors say that coffee and tea are fine in the diet.

Moderation is again the key. Very large amounts of caffeine (five to ten cups of coffee a day) may raise blood sugar. Furthermore, the adverse effects of too much caffeine are often confused with signs of an insulin reaction, or vice versa: anxiety, trembling, and irritability.

What's more, caffeine taken along with glucose—think of a cup of coffee and a danish—has been found to trigger hypoglycemic symptoms such as anxiety and shakiness, even when blood-sugar levels are normal. A group of British investigators, reporting their study at the June 1997 meeting of the American Diabetes Association, say the finding holds for people with and without diabetes, though the experts speculate that those with diabetes may have a more profound reaction and so may want to avoid the combination.

Most people with diabetes can drink alcohol—in moderation, of course. Excessive drinking, however, is likely to wreak havoc with a blood-glucose level, sending it spiraling downward by interfering with the way the liver processes glycogen.

In addition, diabetic drugs known as oral hypoglycemic agents (especially first-generation oral agents—see Chapter 3) may interact with alcohol, causing facial flushing, severe headaches, or dizziness. If that happens, you could ask your doctor to put you on a different oral agent. The new drug might not interact with alcohol, but then again it might—doctors find it impossible to predict who will be affected by which drug. As a result, some people using oral agents find it less aggravating not to drink at all.

If you choose to have an occasional drink (and many people with diabetes do), be aware that alcohol contains empty calories—they have no nutritional value. Those calories must be accounted for when someone is trying to lose or maintain weight.

SUPPLEMENTING YOUR DIET

Dietary supplements—that is, extra vitamins, minerals, and other substances—play a role in diabetes care. Many practitioners recommend a daily multivitamin/mineral supplement, in part because they believe that frequent urination (a hallmark of high blood-sugar levels) may discharge needed nutrients, and in part because they worry that a high-fiber, high-carbohydrate diet may lead to vitamin and mineral binding, which is caused when a food prevents a vitamin or mineral from being absorbed during digestion.

You may have read about chromium, a trace mineral and a common nutrition supplement. Research conducted in China by Richard Anderson, a scientist at the U.S. Department of Agriculture, showed that 500-microgram chromium supplements taken twice a day normalized blood-sugar levels in type 2 diabetes within a couple of months. "These results are preliminary and need to be reproduced in the United States before chromium can be recommended to all people with diabetes," he told *Medical Tribune,* particularly as FDA currently estimates the safe and adequate daily dietary intake of chromium for healthy adults at 50 to 200 micrograms.

Humble vitamin C may also have a role in treating diabetes: In people with type 2 diabetes, vitamin C can improve circulation, says a study published in 1996 in the *Journal of Clinical Investigation.* Improved circulation may help prevent retinopathy, nephropathy, and atherosclerosis, researchers think. There's speculation about vitamin E as well, from researchers at the Joslin Diabetes Center in Falmouth, Massachusetts. They believe that vitamin E, as an antioxidant (a substance that neutralizes damaging molecules called free radicals), may hinder the activation of protein kinase C, a substance thought to contribute to the development of diabetic complications such as vascular damage, neuropathy, hypoglycemia, and diabetic retinopathy.

Eating fish can help prevent coronary heart disease by lowering cholesterol levels, according to numerous studies. However, while fish-oil supplements—specifically omega-3—may help control cholesterol, studies show that they increase blood-sugar levels. Over the long haul, the increased blood-sugar levels would erase any benefit of the fish oil on cardiovascular disease. Today, experts recommend that people with diabetes eat fish, but they advise staying away from fish-oil supplements.

Magnesium deficiency is a common and underrecognized problem with diabetes, according to Alan J. Garber, M.D., of Baylor College of Medicine in Houston, and one that can harm cardiovascular function as well as blood-sugar levels. Two of the most magnesium-rich foods are chocolate and nuts; others are shellfish, legumes, and whole grains. Magnesium chloride supplements are sometimes given to people with poorly controlled diabetes, who are at higher risk of cardiovascular problems.

Zinc deficiency is also a concern for those with diabetes, since zinc is lost with frequent urination and also because of a decreased ability by the intestine to absorb zinc in those with the disease. Here, too, taking supplements or eating foods high in zinc—such as red meat, oysters, and wheat germ—is recommended.

Don't think that you must stick to a traditional healthy diet if you have diabetes. There are plenty of options out there. For example, a carefully planned vegetarian diet can be very healthy. Long-term retrospective studies of vegetarians find that they live longer and healthier lives than their peers who eat the typical American high-protein, high-fat diet. For one thing, vegetarians are less likely to develop heart disease. Legumes, such as beans and peas, which are staples of vegetarian eating plans, are high in fiber and so are thought to help lower blood-cholesterol levels.

The thing to remember is that there are many different foods in the world and many opportunities to mix them in creative, satisfying, and nutritional combinations. Of course, a "good"

Complementary Care: Herbs and Diabetes

There are herbal treatments for diabetes as well, though much of the use of plant treatments for diabetes (as well as the research into their effectiveness) is done overseas in Britain and other areas of Europe and in Asia, where **homeopathic** and **herbal medicine** play a greater role in health care than in the United States. (Homeopathic medicine treats illnesses by using safe, natural substances that stimulate a person's own healing powers while avoiding harmful side effects. Herbal medicine is a healing art that uses plants to prevent and cure illnesses.)

Many herbs are said to help regulate blood-sugar levels; however, not one has been proven to do so. For diabetes, commonly recommended herbs include aloe vera, blueberry leaf, fenugreek, ginkgo, and dandelion.

The American Diabetes Association, for its part, does not recommend any herb for treating diabetes because there is no scientific evidence herbs are helpful. In fact, in some instances they may be harmful. For example, certain herbs may interact poorly with diabetes medications.

If you're thinking about using herbal therapy for your diabetes, remember to talk to your physician, as well as an herbal practitioner. Remember: You should never change your treatment plan for diabetes without first talking to your doctor.

diet or meal plan is not just one that is nutritionally sound—it has to be one that the person with diabetes will eat! In other words, it has to be appetizing to the individual palate. It can—and should—take into account ethnic preferences.

Different ethnic groups historically tend to prefer different types of food. For instance, a healthy lunch for a Caucasian may include a sandwich with whole wheat bread. A sandwich probably wouldn't appeal to a Navajo, who comes from a culture that eats very little wheat flour, but a mutton, bean, and vegetable stew with a corn tortilla might hit the spot. Since diabetes strikes a disproportionate share of some minority groups in this country, people with diabetes shouldn't hesitate to develop (or ask a dietitian to locate) recipes that they find palatable.

It's not our goal to be encyclopedic about nutrition, but we do wish to impress upon you the effect on blood sugar of the foods you choose to eat. There are plenty of sources of more information on fats and carbohydrates, some listed at the end of this book. If you're interested, search these out. The more information you have about your disease, the wiser a medical consumer you'll become, and the better a partner you'll be in your health care.

Exercise and Diabetes

Once you've mastered nutrition, don't think you can sit back and relax. You'd probably be better off slipping on a pair of walking shoes and heading out for a brisk twenty-minute jaunt in the fresh air because exercise is the third crucial element in the treatment of diabetes.

Exercise does many things—it improves a person's state of mind, builds muscle tone, and speeds the process of losing weight. It also gets the circulation going, guards against osteoporosis in women, and lowers the risk of heart disease. Most important for people with diabetes, it lowers blood sugar by making tissues more sensitive to insulin. Twenty minutes of fast walking, for instance, may bring blood glucose down 20 mg/dl.

If you have diabetes and are out of shape or are just new to an exercise regimen, you should check with a health care practitioner before launching into an exercise program. A physician can give you the details about the optimum heartbeat rate for someone your age, weight, and overall physical condition.

Since exercise lowers blood sugar, people with type 1 diabetes will initially need medical assistance in determining how to adjust food intake and insulin doses on their new exercise plans. In fact, people who are insulin dependent—or those with type 2 diabetes who are on oral agents—need to exercise a few precautions before exercising their limbs.

For example, if you have type 1, you may need to eat before, during, or after exercising to compensate for the anticipated drop in blood sugar. Many exercisers who have diabetes carry a small sugary snack in case blood-sugar levels fall too low. If you're insulin dependent and exercise vigorously, you should inform the people you exercise with and teach them about the symptoms of hypoglycemia (dangerously low blood sugar). Wearing a bracelet or necklace or carrying a wallet card that identifies you as insulin dependent is an extra measure of precaution.

Most authorities in the field recommend a three-times-a-week program of walking, swimming, jogging, bicycling, aerobics, rowing, hiking, cross-country skiing—whatever you can handle, as long as it gets your heart pumping for twenty to thirty minutes. These exercises, called **aerobic exercises,** build cardiovascular fitness.

Exercise buffs will tell you that it's important to warm up before exercising and to cool down afterward. Look for flexibility exercises—stretching and bending—to help you loosen up your joints and prepare your muscles for the work ahead. Flexibility exercises reduce the chance of injuring muscles.

Frequent exercise is essential because the benefit of exercise on insulin efficiency does not last very long. People who are trying to lose weight might do well to remember that the more often they exercise, the more calories they burn. Exercising three or more times a week can help people lose weight faster.

Research from Harvard Medical School has found that regular vigorous exercise—the kind that works up a sweat—may protect people against developing diabetes. In their study of 87,253 women from 1980 to 1988, the researchers found that compared with women who did not exercise, women who exercised vigorously at least once a week lowered by one-third the risk of developing type 2 diabetes.

By vigorous exercise, we mean stepping up the intensity while walking, playing tennis, jogging, swimming, hiking, bicycling, and the like so that you work up a sweat. "Strenuous" is another word researchers use to describe activities that make you perspire.

Even a simple routine of "power" walking or swimming several days a week can help. And there's more good news—the Harvard study showed the benefit of exercise held true whether the women were obese, moderately overweight, or not overweight and was beneficial regardless of family history of diabetes.

Research has since confirmed the same phenomenon in men. One study, reported in the *Journal of the American Medical Association* in 1992, found that the more frequently the men exercised, the less likely they were to develop type 2 diabetes, even in the face of other risk factors, such as smoking, high blood pressure, and obesity! Men who worked up a sweat five or more times a week had 42 percent less risk of developing diabetes than those who exercised less than once a week. Men who worked out two to four times per week reduced the risk 38 percent, and those who broke a sweat once a week reduced the risk 23 percent.

There are some caveats, however. People with diabetes need to know when not to exercise. This includes times when blood-sugar levels are over 300 mg/dl, when insulin or oral agents are peaking, when ketones are present in urine, or when they are ill (even with a cold), injured, or experiencing feelings of pain, tingling, dizziness, numbness, or nausea. Nor should someone with diabetes exercise on his feet when he has a foot injury.

Exercise might exacerbate a blister, bruise, or cut, resulting in an infection or an ulcer.

Sad to say, too, that some people with diabetes can't exercise because their disease has already progressed too far. In particular, regular physical activity may not be possible for people who have developed severe diabetic complications. One study that looked at 837 hospitalized people with insulin-treated type 2 diabetes found that 69 percent had at least one complication that precluded vigorous exercise or demanded special precautionary measures if exercise were to be attempted. Granted, those folks were hospitalized and so had a more severe form of diabetes than many of their peers. But the lesson is clear: People with diabetes must begin exercise programs as early in the course of their disease as possible, before it's too late to reap exercise's many benefits.

Foot Care

Exercise helps maintain your health, but it also helps if you're in good health when you start your regimen, which brings us to a related area of self-care: proper care of the feet.

For starters, examine your feet every day for even minor problems, such as cuts, corns, bruises, and blisters. If undetected, any one of these seemingly simple problems can lead to a major infection and, in extreme cases, gangrene. Diabetic foot disease is the cause of 20 percent of hospitalizations for people with diabetes, and, as we mentioned in Chapter 4, diabetes-related amputations account for half of all lower-limb amputations performed in the United States. Fortunately, there are ways to prevent yourself from becoming one of those statistics. Here's how:

- Inspect and wash your feet daily in warm (not hot) water; blot to dry, and do not rub between the toes. Use a moisturizing cream (but not between the toes).

- Change shoes twice daily. Wear leather shoes with large toe boxes, such as soft leather jogging shoes.

- Wear clean cotton or wool socks that are the proper size for your feet.

- Don't use hot water bottles, heating pads, or heat lamps near your feet.

- Don't cross your legs when sitting (it reduces circulation in the legs), and don't wear garters.

- Don't cut your toenails—file them so that they are straight across. Slightly round the corners by filing them diagonally. Toenails that are too short or that are clipped incorrectly can become ingrown, which may lead to infection. Filing rather than cutting also eliminates the risk of cutting the skin along with the nail.

- Don't use chemical agents to remove corns or calluses, and don't use inserts or pads without checking with your health care practitioner.

- Don't wear new shoes for more than an hour at one time until they are broken in, and don't wear shoes without socks.

- Never go barefoot outdoors! Sandals and open-toed shoes are invitations to problems, too.

- Get your feet tested annually with a monofilament, a simple nylon device that we talked about in Chapter 4. Self-administered foot tests may also soon be available to people with diabetes to complement professional foot assessments.

Dental Care

In addition to the feet, the teeth and gums also require special attention. Uncontrolled diabetes seems to increase the risk of gum disease (a major cause of tooth loss) and leads to more cavities.

Regular dental self-care (brushing and flossing teeth) and regular dental checkups are important in people with high blood sugar. Watch for the signs of gum disease, which include bleeding or swollen gums, receding gums, and loose teeth, and report them to your dentist immediately.

Smoking

And speaking of the mouth—one thing you should never put in it is a cigarette. Everyone knows that cigarette smoking increases the risk of heart disease and lung cancer. Smoking has those negative impacts on people with diabetes, and it tacks on others: Studies suggest that insulin users who smoke require 15 to 20 percent more insulin than nonsmokers.

But the biggest reason to give up smoking is that it increases the risk of diabetic complications such as cardiovascular and kidney disease by accelerating small-blood-vessel damage. Recent research also shows that the sugars in tobacco—which enter the body through cigarette smoke—undergo chemical reactions in the body, ultimately forming clumps of cholesterol and other substances that stick to and clog artery walls. People with diabetes already have higher rates of cardiovascular and kidney complications—why compound the risk?

Self-Care Through the Ages

Certain situations also affect diabetes self-care. Interestingly enough, these pertain to certain times of life: youth and adolescence, the childbearing years, and advanced age.

CHILDREN AND DIABETES

As with adults, the goal in treating children with diabetes is to keep blood sugar within normal ranges and to prevent dangerous short-term complications such as hypoglycemia and ketoacidosis. And of course, good exercise and eating habits must be part of the treatment plan.

Children can practice self-care themselves once they get to be of school age. They can be taught to recognize the symptoms of hypoglycemia and ketoacidosis, understand the fundamentals of meal planning, and even self-monitor their blood glucose.

Very young children obviously require extra care from Mom and Dad, and even older kids still need supervision to ensure that they balance exercise with food intake or that they don't overindulge in sweets with friends. Teenagers, who are often fiercely independent (or try to be), may resent having to practice a somewhat rigid meal and medicine routine. They may try to take shortcuts, such as neglecting their SMBG. However, the hormonal changes of puberty can make blood-sugar levels less predictable, meaning SMBG is required more rather than less often. Parents and doctors may find that they may have to work out some type of compromise with teenagers, trading extra control in one area (SMBG, for example) with more flexibility in another (such as type of food eaten).

There are many excellent sources of diabetes information designed just for young people—both children and teenagers—and we list some at the end of this chapter. Use them! And remember: It's never too early to teach self-care—or to practice it.

PREGNANCY AND DIABETES

Women with diabetes who plan to become pregnant should first get blood-sugar levels under control, using the strategies

Eating Disorders and Diabetes

When you think of how television and magazines portray thin as beautiful, it's easy to understand why eating disorders are a growing problem in the United States. More than 8 million Americans suffer from conditions such as anorexia nervosa (eating very little and purging to lose weight), bulimia (binging and then purging to maintain weight), and binge-eating disorder (binging and weight gain), which center around an obsession with food and body weight.

The risk for eating disorders seems to be greater for people with diabetes than for the general population, in part because dietary restrictions may spark a preoccupation with food and weight that can develop into an eating disorder. People with diabetes may also try too hard to control what they eat, feeling that their lives are out of control in other ways. Diabetes also often masks a developing eating disorder, with preoccupation passed off as careful disease control instead of a growing obsession.

Eating disorders are especially dangerous for people with diabetes, because food restriction and binging can bring on wide swings in blood-sugar levels, from hypoglycemia to hyperglycemia, both of which can lead to complications and, in the worst case, death. Treating such conditions is difficult and involves professional therapy and sometimes medical care. If you or a loved one has an eating disorder, seek immediate care.

we've discussed in this book. Well-managed diabetes reduces the risk of complications during pregnancy, but pregnancy requires extra effort and attention to blood sugar, calorie intake, nutritional balance, and exercise. Even with extra care there are potential problems, such as premature birth, an abnormally large baby (caused by the effects of high blood sugar on the fetus), a difficult birth, or an infant born with respiratory problems, low blood calcium, jaundice, or an infection.

The insulin doses and food required to control diabetes change during pregnancy: A woman may need nearly three times more insulin by the time she is ready to deliver. The goal, as with all insulin therapy, is to keep blood sugar as close to normal ranges as possible.

Most women are able to control diabetes during pregnancy through diet and exercise, although a few go on to use human insulin. (Oral agents cannot be used during pregnancy.) Self-monitoring of blood glucose is mandatory.

All women with diabetes can expect to undergo additional tests during the course of pregnancy. They might include fetal tests, such as the **alpha fetoprotein** test, to check for possible spinal defects. **Ultrasound** tests check the health and development of the fetus and estimate its weight and size (information that determines whether the baby can be delivered through the vagina or whether a cesarean delivery may be required). Other tests for pregnant women may include an electrocardiogram to check heart condition, kidney-function tests, urine-ketone tests, and frequent eye exams to watch for diabetic retinopathy. Women who have moderate to severe retinopathy may need to be examined as often as once a month because pregnancy speeds the course of this disease.

On the whole, women with diabetes or gestational diabetes need frequent medical attention, with an eye on controlling blood sugar and pregnancy-related complications. After the pregnancy, the treatment returns to that used before the pregnancy. Women are encouraged to breast-feed their babies (though that may require additional insulin) since it's good for the health of both mother and child.

Another area of concern after pregnancy is the use of oral contraception. Many—but not all—oral contraceptives can provoke type 2 diabetes in women with a history of gestational diabetes. Women who have had gestational diabetes during a prior pregnancy must carefully select their oral contraceptives with the help of their practitioners.

AGING AND DIABETES

Blood-glucose levels begin to increase in everyone in their fifties and sixties. And while people may not develop diabetes per se, they may develop impaired glucose tolerance, or slight elevations in blood sugar. This may be a function of aging, and it may be related to insulin resistance associated with being overweight.

Either way, even slight increases in blood sugar put people at greater risk of cardiovascular problems, meaning that the elderly need to pay special attention to diet and exercise.

Food may play a role in preventing or slowing the onset of glucose intolerance. In one recent study, Dutch researchers found that 60 percent of people ages sixty-four to eighty-seven who regularly ate fish—usually an ounce a day—were less likely to develop glucose intolerance than people who didn't eat fish.

Elderly people with full-fledged diabetes may have difficulty adhering to their regimens for unique reasons. Vision problems or decreased manual dexterity may make it more difficult to use syringes or glucose meters accurately. Exercise plans become more difficult to maintain. Kidney function also declines with age, which means the elderly face a greater risk of kidney complications. Of course, not all older people with diabetes have these problems—many are robust and healthy. But to make the task of self-care easier on the elderly, some doctors recommend more frequent blood tests, a simple meal plan, and office visits every three months to check for eye and foot problems.

Practicing Prevention

Not all practitioners practice prevention. Recent reports suggest that primary care physicians are not very reliable about performing preventive exams in patients with diabetes. According to a representative from the Centers for Disease Control and

Prevention (CDC), self-reports from more than 1,000 primary care physicians suggest not all doctors are up to date on recommended tests and examinations. In addition, the CDC has found that people with type 1 diabetes generally receive more preventive services than do those with type 2. Apparently, type 2 diabetes is still seen as less serious than type 1 diabetes—a problem in attitude that we discussed in the opening pages of this book.

Recommended prevention services include quarterly blood-pressure measurements, twice-a-year foot examinations, annual exams for diabetic retinopathy, regular inspection of gums and teeth (a relatively new recommendation), and certain tests: the **glycosylated hemoglobin,** urine protein, and creatinine clearance tests.

One of the newest and most important lab tests is the glycosylated hemoglobin, or glycohemoglobin. The glycosylated hemoglobin test, also called the **hemoglobin A_{1C} test,** measures the number of glucose molecules ("glyco") attached to hemoglobin, a substance within the red blood cells. This gives a reading of the average sugar level over the previous two to three months in contrast to a blood-glucose test, which gives a reading of blood glucose at only one particular moment in time.

The glycosylated hemoglobin test is one of the most important ways of measuring overall diabetes control. Performed every three months or so, it shows you and your doctor how well your treatment regimen is working by telling where your glucose levels have been, on average, for the last two months.

The test also shows if the data gathered from SMBG are reasonably accurate. Unfortunately, the Agency for Health Care Policy and Research reports more than 40 percent of people with diabetes who use insulin (and 30 percent who do not) do not have this test every year.

The following are some of the most common laboratory tests. Certain of these tests should be performed several times a year; others should be done yearly (or less often, depending upon the severity of your disease).

- *Cholesterol test* (sometimes called a lipid profile). This is actually a series of tests that measure lipids, or fatty substances, in the blood. These tests include (1) total serum cholesterol, (2) HDL cholesterol, and (3) triglycerides. They are performed to determine a person's total cholesterol, LDL-cholesterol level, and triglyceride levels. High levels of these increase the risk of heart disease and often are signals of inadequate diabetes control, as we mentioned earlier in this chapter.

- *Urinalysis.* This screens for urinary-tract infections, which, if allowed unchecked, may lead to kidney damage.

- *Creatinine clearance.* This test measures the filtering capacity of the kidneys, and thus is used to monitor deterioration of the kidneys. It requires a blood test and a "twenty-four-hour urine specimen"—that is, all the urine a person produced in twenty-four hours.

- *Microalbuminuria.* This test also reflects early kidney changes and often requires a twenty-four-hour urine specimen.

Many other tests may be done depending upon the severity of your disease and may include an electrocardiogram, an angiogram, or a thyroid function test. Many of these are geared toward detecting or evaluating a diabetic complication.

You may have noticed that a blood-glucose test isn't included on this list. At first glance, it might seem that a blood-glucose test should be a part of the battery of office tests. In fact, guidelines set by the American College of Physicians in 1990 call for the use of home glucose testing as a substitute for routine testing in a doctor's office.

If you think about it, that makes sense. Since people with diabetes can self-monitor blood glucose with any of the simple home testing kits, why pay for a blood-sugar reading in a doctor's office when it can—and, some say, should—be done at home? Just be sure to bring your notebook with your SMBG results to the doctor's office, so she can see the most recent blood-sugar levels.

Self-care boils down to your taking responsibility for the treatment of your disease. Although you will work closely with your doctor, it's ultimately up to you to make the commitment to control your disease, instead of letting it control you. Managing diabetes properly takes commitment and understanding.

Hopefully, you've found some of the information you need to gain that understanding in these pages. We hope you also find the motivation it takes to put that information into action, working toward your own good health.

Informational and Mutual-Aid Groups

American Association of Diabetes Educators
100 W. Monroe St., 4th Floor
Chicago, IL 60603-1901
312-424-2426
www.aadenet.org

American Diabetes Association, National Center
1660 Duke St.
Alexandria, VA 22314
800-232-3472 (check your phone book for local chapters)
www.diabetes.org

American Dietetic Association
216 W. Jackson Blvd., Suite 800
Chicago, IL 60606-6995
312-899-0040
www.eatright.org

Juvenile Diabetes Foundation International
120 Wall St.
New York, NY 10005
800-223-1138
212-889-7575
www.jdfcure.org

National Diabetes Information Clearinghouse
1 Information Way
Bethesda, MD 20892-3560
301-654-3327
www.niddk.nih.gov/health/diabetes/ndic.htm

Glossary

Absorbency   How quickly insulin takes effect.

Acarbose   Oral hypoglycemic agent used to lower blood-sugar levels.

Acetohexamide   Oral hypoglycemic agent used to lower blood-sugar levels.

Acetones   See **Ketones.**

Acute   Referring to a condition that develops quickly and is intense, and then may ease after a short time; sharp or severe.

Adult-onset diabetes   Term once used for type 2 diabetes.

Aerobic exercise   Steady activity that gets your heart pumping and makes you work up a sweat.

Aldose reductase   Enzyme thought to play a role in triggering diabetic complications.

Aldose reductase inhibitors   Class of drugs that block the action of the enzyme aldose reductase.

Algorithm   A simple mathematical chart that can serve as a guide for determining how many units of insulin to take and when to take them, depending upon blood-sugar levels.

Alpha fetoprotein   Test that screens for possible spinal defects in an unborn baby.

Angiogram   X-ray that locates blockages in large blood vessels.

Antibodies Substances created by the immune system to destroy antigens. In an autoimmune disease, antibodies may destroy a body's own cells.

Antigens Proteins or enzymes capable of stimulating an immune response.

Arteriosclerosis Hardening of the arteries.

Artery Blood vessel that carries blood away from the heart.

Atherosclerosis Form of arteriosclerosis in which inner walls of arteries thicken due to deposits of fat, cholesterol, and other substances.

Autoimmune Term used to describe what happens when the body's immune system attacks itself.

Autonomic neuropathy Damage to the nerves that control bodily functions such as the digestive system, urinary tract, and cardiovascular system.

Background retinopathy Mild, early form of the disease of retinal blood vessels.

Beef-derived insulin Insulin obtained from the pancreas of a steer.

Beta cells Cells in the pancreas that produce and secrete insulin into the bloodstream when blood-sugar levels rise.

Blood glucose Blood sugar, the body's primary source of energy.

Blood-glucose meter Device to test blood-sugar levels.

Blood pressure Force of blood against the walls of blood vessels.

Borderline diabetes Another term for impaired glucose tolerance.

Brittle diabetes Dramatic swings in blood-sugar levels.

Bromocriptine Drug that increases insulin sensitivity and suppresses appetite and enables obese people with type 2 diabetes to improve glycemic control by losing weight.

Bypass surgery   Method of rerouting blood around obstructions in a blood vessel.

Capillaries   Tiny blood vessels that carry blood between the smallest arteries and the smallest veins.

Carbohydrate   One of the three basic sources of energy in food; found in grains, vegetables, and fruits.

Cardiac   Pertaining to the heart.

Cardiovascular   Pertaining to the heart and blood vessels.

Cataract   Clouding of the lens of the eye or of its surrounding transparent membrane that obstructs the passage of light.

Catheter   Tubular medical device for insertion into canals, vessels, or body cavities, usually to allow injection or withdrawal of fluids.

Chlorpropamide   Oral hypoglycemic agent used to lower blood-sugar levels.

Cholesterol   Fatlike substance found in meat and dairy products and also manufactured by the body.

Chronic   Referring to a condition or disease that develops slowly and persists for a long period of time.

Closed-loop pump   Implantable insulin pump.

Combination therapy   Treatment of type 2 diabetes using a combination of two different medications.

Complex carbohydrate   Carbohydrate made from more complex chains of sugar that are digested more slowly and raise blood-sugar levels less rapidly than simple carbohydrate.

Continuous subcutaneous insulin infusion (CSII)   Form of intensive insulin therapy using an insulin pump.

Conventional therapy   In diabetes, use of insulin to keep blood-sugar levels within certain target ranges; less stringent than tight control.

Dawn phenomenon Sudden increase in blood sugar that occurs in early morning.

Degree Intensity of effect or the activity insulin creates.

Diabetes mellitus Disease resulting from the body's inability to produce or use insulin, resulting in high blood-sugar levels.

Diabetic coma Another term for ketoacidosis, or dangerously high blood-sugar levels, which can cause coma and death.

Dialysis Use of a machine to filter wastes from blood after kidneys have failed.

Diet therapy Use of an eating plan to lower blood-sugar levels.

Duration The length of time of the effect or the activity insulin creates.

Epinephrine Naturally occurring hormone that works to keep insulin and blood-sugar levels balanced; also called adrenaline.

Euglycemia Normal levels of blood sugar.

Fasting Not eating for three or more hours.

Fasting plasma glucose test Measurement of blood-sugar level before the first meal of the day, usually twelve hours after eating.

Fat One of the three basic sources of energy in food; found in dairy products, meat, fish, nuts, oils, and some vegetables.

Fiber Indigestible material in grains, vegetables, and fruits; see **insoluble fiber** and **soluble fiber**.

Fructose Sugar in fruits, vegetables, and honey.

Gangrene Death of body tissues due to a loss of blood supply.

Gestational diabetes Diabetes that develops or is discovered in a woman during pregnancy.

Glimepiride Oral hypoglycemic agent used to lower blood-sugar levels.

Glipizide   Oral hypoglycemic agent used to lower blood-sugar levels.

Glomeruli   Tuftlike structures composed of blood vessels or nerve fibers.

Glucagon   Naturally occurring hormone (produced by the pancreas) that helps regulate blood-sugar levels.

Glucose   Sugar; the body's primary energy source.

Glyburide   Oral hypoglycemic agent used to lower blood-sugar levels.

Glycemia   Blood-sugar level.

Glycemic   Pertaining to blood-sugar level.

Glycemic control   Overall control of blood-sugar levels.

Glycemic index   Scientific measurement of the effect of different foods on blood-sugar levels.

Glycogen   Storage form of glucose.

Glycosylated hemoglobin   Test that measures the number of glucose molecules attached to hemoglobin, a substance within the red blood cells; used to estimate average blood-sugar levels over the prior two months.

Hemoglobin A_{1C} test   Term sometimes used for the glycosylated hemoglobin test.

Hemorrhage   A loss of a large amount of blood in a short period of time, either outside or inside the body.

Herbal medicine   Healing art that uses plants to prevent and cure illnesses.

High blood pressure   Increase in blood pressure above normal levels; also called hypertension.

High-density lipoprotein (HDL)   "Good" cholesterol; the substance that escorts excess cholesterol out of the body.

Homeopathic medicine Healing art that treats illnesses by using safe, natural medicines that stimulate a person's own healing powers while avoiding harmful side effects.

Human insulin Insulin manufactured to be chemically identical to the insulin normally produced by the body.

Hypercholesterolemia High levels of cholesterol in the blood.

Hyperglycemia High blood-sugar levels.

Hyperinsulinemia High levels of insulin in the blood.

Hyperlipidemia High levels of fatty substances in the blood.

Hyperosmolar coma Dangerous dehydration and/or loss of consciousness caused by high blood-sugar levels; differs chemically from ketoacidosis.

Hypertension High blood pressure.

Hypertriglyceridemia High levels of triglycerides in the blood.

Hypoglycemia Low blood-sugar levels.

Hypoglycemic unawareness Occurs when people with low blood-sugar levels do not experience or detect the warning signals of hypoglycemia.

Iatrogenic Caused by medical treatment.

Immunosuppressive drugs Drugs used to stop the immune system from attacking some substance.

Immunotherapy Method of treatment used to stop the immune system from attacking some substance.

Impaired glucose tolerance (IGT) Blood-sugar levels higher than normal but not high enough to be diagnosed as diabetes.

Implantable pump A small device inserted under the skin that pumps insulin into the body at specified intervals.

Impotence   Loss of male sexual functioning.

Increased risk for diabetes   Term applied to someone at increased risk of developing diabetes in the future.

Injection site   Area where insulin is injected.

Insoluble fiber   Indigestible material found in certain grains, vegetables, and fruits that absorbs water but doesn't dissolve in it.

Insulin   Hormone produced in pancreas that enables the body to use sugar for energy.

Insulin allergy   Adverse reaction to insulin.

Insulin-dependent diabetes   Term once used for type 1 diabetes.

Insulin pen   Device shaped like a pen that is used to inject insulin.

Insulin pump   Battery-operated device that pumps insulin into the body at specified intervals.

Insulin reaction   Low blood sugar caused by too much insulin, not enough food, or too much exercise.

Insulin resistance   Term applied when insulin is produced by the body but is not being used efficiently.

Insulin shock   Hypoglycemic shock caused by an overdose of insulin, a decreased intake of food, or too much exercise; characterized by trembling, sweating, nervousness, irritability, hunger, hallucination, numbness, and pallor.

Intensive therapy   Type of diabetes therapy that strives for tight control of blood-sugar levels within certain narrow targets; also called tight control.

Intermediate-acting insulin   Insulin that works more quickly than long-acting insulin but not as quickly as short-acting insulin.

Intraocular lens   Artificial lens implanted in eye.

Islets, or **islets of Langerhans** Clusters of cells in the pancreas that include the beta cells, which make insulin.

Juvenile diabetes Term once used for type 1 diabetes.

Ketoacidosis In diabetes, a dangerous condition caused by very high blood sugars, dehydration, and high blood levels of ketones.

Ketones Toxic acids produced by the body when it uses fat instead of glucose for energy.

Ketonuria Ketones in urine.

Ketosis Ketones in blood.

Lactic acidosis A life-threatening buildup of acid in the blood that may develop in people with heart, kidney, or liver disease.

Lactose Sugar found in dairy products.

Lancet Special needle used for pricking the finger to get a drop of blood; used in self-monitoring of blood glucose.

Latent diabetes See **impaired glucose tolerance.**

Lente insulin Intermediate-acting insulin.

Lipid Fat and/or fatty substance.

Lispro insulin Short-acting insulin.

Long-acting insulin Insulin that takes effect slowly and works for a long period of time.

Low-density lipoprotein (LDL) "Bad" cholesterol; substance that aids in deposit of fats on artery and cell walls.

Macrovascular Pertaining to the large blood vessels.

Macula Area of the retina responsible for sharp, fine vision.

Macular edema Swelling of the area near the center of retina.

Markers In diabetes, genetic signposts on a cell that indicate whether diabetes will develop.

Maturity-onset diabetes   Term once used for type 2 diabetes.

Maturity-onset diabetes of the young   Term sometimes applied for type 2 diabetes in children and adolescents.

Metabolism   Process of converting food into energy to power the body.

Metformin   Oral hypoglycemic agent used to lower blood-sugar levels.

Microaneurysm   Small swelling on small blood vessels.

Microvascular   Pertaining to the small blood vessels.

Mixed-split regimen   Diabetes treatment in which mixtures of intermediate-acting insulin and short-acting insulin are given before breakfast and dinner.

Monofilament   Tool used to test for nerve damage in the feet.

Monounsaturated fat   Fat that may protect against vascular disease by lowering LDL cholesterol and raising HDL cholesterol.

Nephropathy   Kidney disease or damage leading to kidney failure.

Neuropathic ulcer   An area of infected tissue that is difficult to heal.

Neuropathy   Nerve damage resulting in severe pain or loss of feeling.

Non-insulin-dependent diabetes   Term once used for type 2 diabetes.

Nonketotic coma   Term sometimes used for hyperosmolar coma.

Normoglycemia   Normal levels of blood sugar.

NPH insulin   Intermediate-acting insulin.

Onset   When referring to insulin, how quickly insulin takes effect.

Ophthalmologist   A physician who specializes in the eye.

Oral glucose-tolerance test   Series of blood tests used to determine how the body reacts to glucose over a period of several hours.

Oral hypoglycemic agent   Drug used to lower blood sugar in people with type 2 diabetes; also called an oral agent.

Oral therapy   Diabetes therapy that uses oral hypoglycemic agents.

Orthostatic hypotension   Sudden drop in blood pressure when a person gets up after reclining.

Pancreas   Gland located behind the stomach that produces insulin, glucagon, and other hormones and enzymes.

Peripheral neuropathy   Nerve damage in hands, legs, and feet.

Photocoagulation   Use of laser beam to sear leaking blood vessels shut.

Plasma   The liquid component of the blood.

Polydipsia   Long-lasting thirst; symptom of diabetes.

Polyphagia   Unsatisfied hunger; symptom of diabetes.

Polyunsaturated fat   Fatty acids that may reduce LDL cholesterol.

Polyuria   Frequent urination; symptom of diabetes.

Pork-derived insulin   Insulin made from pork pancreas.

Postprandial   After a meal.

Potential abnormality of glucose   Term applied to people who have a close relative with type 1 diabetes or people with islet cell antibodies.

Previous abnormality of glucose tolerance   Term applied to people who have experienced impaired glucose tolerance in the past but have no sign of abnormal glucose metabolism now.

Primary failure   Situation in which an oral hypoglycemic agent fails to lower blood-sugar levels.

Proliferative retinopathy   Advanced disease of retinal blood vessels.

Protein   One of the three basic sources of energy in food found in fish, meat, eggs, and, in lesser amounts, grains and legumes.

PZI   Protamine zinc insulin; a long-acting insulin.

Reaction denial   Situation in which a person with diabetes does not admit he is having an insulin reaction, usually because blood-glucose levels in the brain are too low.

Rebound   Return to high blood sugar after levels had been lowered.

Receptors   Structures that serve as gateways to the cell, allowing insulin and other chemicals to enter.

Receptor sites   Places where receptors are located.

Regular insulin   Short-acting insulin.

Renal   Pertaining to kidneys.

Repaglinide   Oral hypoglycemic agent used to lower blood-sugar levels.

Retina   Light-sensing surface on the rear wall of the eye.

Retinopathy   Disease of retinal blood vessels.

Saturated fat   Fat from animal sources that contributes to high cholesterol.

Secondary diabetes   Term used to describe a host of other conditions that can give rise to diabetes. In many such cases, the diabetes is a secondary condition that results from another disease, medication, or chemical. Among the causes of secondary diabetes are pancreatic diseases (especially chronic pancreatitis in alcoholics), hormonal abnormalities (including ones that result from the administration of steroids), insulin-receptor disorders, drug- or chemical-induced diabetes, and certain genetic syndromes.

Secondary failure   Situation in which an oral hypoglycemic agent that once lowered blood-sugar levels suddenly stops working.

Self-monitoring of blood glucose (SMBG)   Technique in which people with diabetes keep track of their day-to-day blood-sugar levels.

Semilente insulin   Short-acting insulin.

Semisynthetic   Term applied to human insulin that has been made by chemical modification of pork-derived insulin.

Short-acting insulin   Insulin that takes effect quickly.

Simple carbohydrate   Carbohydrate that can be quickly converted to glucose during digestion.

Simple sugar   Simple carbohydrate.

SMBG   Abbreviation for self-monitoring of blood glucose.

Soluble fiber   Indigestible material in certain grains, vegetables, and fruits that dissolves in water, turning into a thick, gelatinous mass.

Sorbitol   Sweetener used in diet foods; also, a sugar alcohol produced by the body during the conversion of glucose.

Species   Term referring to the source of insulin, whether beef derived, pork derived, or synthetically manufactured.

Standard therapy   In diabetes, use of insulin to keep blood-sugar levels within certain target ranges; less stringent than tight control.

Stroke   Blockage in the circulation of blood to the brain.

Subcutaneous   Below the skin but above muscle.

Sucrose   Simple sugar.

Sulfonylureas   Oral hypoglycemic agent used to lower blood-sugar levels.

Synthetic   Insulin produced in the laboratory through a recombinant DNA process.

Tight control   Type of diabetes therapy that strives for tight control of blood-sugar levels within certain narrow targets; also called intensive therapy.

Tolazamide   Oral hypoglycemic agent used to lower blood-sugar levels.

Tolbutamide   Oral hypoglycemic agent used to lower blood-sugar levels.

Total serum cholesterol   Measurement of overall level of cholesterol in the blood.

Toxemia   Presence of bacterial poison in the bloodstream.

Triglyceride   A compound made up of fatty acid and glycerol; a storage form of fat.

Troglitazone   Oral hypoglycemic agent used to lower blood-sugar levels.

Type 1 diabetes   Type of diabetes in which the body loses the capacity to produce insulin; once called type I diabetes, insulin-dependent diabetes, and juvenile-onset diabetes.

Type 2 diabetes   Type of diabetes in which the body produces some insulin that is ineffective. It usually appears after age forty and is associated with obesity; once called type II diabetes, non-insulin-dependent diabetes, and adult-onset diabetes.

Ultralente insulin   Long-acting insulin.

Ultrasound   Test that uses sound waves to create a picture of organs and structures deep inside the body; used to check the health and development of a fetus.

Unsaturated fats   Fatty acids that are liquid at room temperature and that may reduce cholesterol levels.

Vascular   Pertaining to blood vessels.

Very low-density lipoprotein (VLDL)   A form of fat known as triglyceride.

Vitrectomy   Surgical removal of the vitreous humor from the eye.

Vitreous hemorrhage   Major hemorrhage in the eye that affects sight.

Vitreous humor   Clear gelatinous material in the center of the eye.

Suggested Reading

American Diabetes Association. *The American Diabetes Association Complete Guide to Diabetes: The Ultimate Home Diabetes Reference.* Alexandria, Va.: American Diabetes Association, 1997.

American Diabetes Association. *Clinical Practice Recommendations, 1998.* Supplement to *Diabetes Care* 21 (Jan. 1998).

American Diabetes Association. *Diabetes A to Z: What You Need to Know About Diabetes Simply Put.* Alexandria, Va.: American Diabetes Association, 1998.

Beaser, Richard S., et al. *The Joslin Guide to Diabetes: A Program for Managing Your Treatment.* New York: Fireside, 1995.

Court, Simon, and Bill Lamb, eds. *Childhood and Adolescent Diabetes.* New York: John Wiley & Sons, 1997.

Dorland's Illustrated Medical Dictionary, 28th ed. Philadelphia: W.B. Saunders, 1994.

Fong, Donald S., and Robin Demi Ross. *The Diabetes Eye Care Sourcebook.* Chicago: Contemporary Books, 1998.

Krall, Leo P., M.D., and Richard S. Beaser, M.D. *Joslin Diabetes Manual,* 12th ed. Philadelphia: Lea & Febiger, 1992.

Lowe, Ernest, and Gary Arsham. *Diabetes: A Guide to Living Well.* Minneapolis: Chronimed, 1997.

Schade, David S., M.D., et al. *101 Tips for Improving Your Blood Sugar: A Project of the American Diabetes Association.* Alexandria, Va.: American Diabetes Association, 1995.

Index

Acarbose, 91
Acetohexamide, 89
Acetones, 113
Adult-onset diabetes. *See* Type 2
  diabetes
African-Americans, 21, 138
Aging, 22, 188–89
Alcohol, 172–73
Aldose reductase inhibitors, 124
Algorithm, 46–47
Allergies
  to insulin, 42
  to sulfonylureas, 90
Alpha-glucosidase inhibitors, 88, 91
American Diabetes Association, 2,
  32, 56, 72
  diet guidelines, 157
  treatment plan, 35–36
Amputations, 7, 104, 138
Angiogram, 139
Antibodies, 10, 67, 68
Antigens, HLA, 67
Antioxidants, 174
Anxiety, 108, 110
Appetite, suppression of, 93
Arms, loss of feeling in, 7
Arteriosclerosis, 128, 129, 132, 163
Asians, 21
Aspartame, 165
Aspirin, 133

Atherosclerosis, 81, 162
Autoimmunity, 9–10

Becaplermin gel, 140
Beef-derived insulin, 39, 41, 43
Bernstein, Richard K., 158
Beta blockers, 18
Beta cells, 10, 13, 80, 88
  transplanting, 72–73, 101
Biermann, June, 82
Biguanides, 90–91
Bladder, 128
Blindness, 104, 119
Blood-glucose levels, 23–24, 104
  and exercise, 87, 178
  and food intake, 84
  lowering, 88–95
  self-monitoring, 47, 110,
    142–55
  target ranges, 85, 105
Blood-glucose meters, 47, 143,
  150–54
Blood pressure, 17–18, 22, 86, 130
  and glucose tolerance, 17
  and nephropathy, 128
  and retinopathy, 126
Blood-sugar
  high, 3, 5–6, 10, 23, 80. *See also*
    Hyperglycemia
  low. *See* Hypoglycemia